Natural Treatments

for

Genital Herpes, Cold Sores and Shingles

A Review of the Scientific and Medical Literature

Second Edition   **By John W Hill**

ISBN-13: 978-1-884979-05-7
ISBN-10: 1-884979-05-x

Library of Congress Control No.: 2007908754

BISAC Subject Headings:

HEA032000	**HEALTH & FITNESS** / Alternative Therapies
HEA039070	**HEALTH & FITNESS** / Diseases / Genitourinary & STDs
HEA020000	**HEALTH & FITNESS** / Reference
HEA024000	**HEALTH & FITNESS** / Women's Health
HEA015000	**HEALTH & FITNESS** / Men's Health
HEA039020	**HEALTH & FITNESS** / Diseases / AIDS & HIV
HEA039040	**HEALTH & FITNESS** / Diseases / Contagious
HEA042000	**HEALTH & FITNESS** / Sexuality
HEA023000	**HEALTH & FITNESS** / Vitamins
MED004000	**MEDICAL** / Alternative Medicine
MED017000	**MEDICAL** / Dermatology
MED022000	**MEDICAL** / Diseases
MED040000	**MEDICAL** / Holistic Medicine
MED022090	**MEDICAL** / Infectious Diseases

Published by: Clear Springs Press, LLC
            Yelm, WA   U.S.A.
http://www.clspress.com/contact.html

Please note, it is extremely important to obtain an accurate diagnosis before trying to find a cure. Many diseases and conditions share common symptoms: if you treat yourself for the wrong illness or for a specific symptom of a complex disease, you may delay more effective treatment of a serious underlying problem. The greatest danger in self-treatment may be incorrect self-diagnosis. You should consult with a doctor to obtain a correct diagnosis and to discuss treatment options, including the options described in this document.

Where to Order this Book

(1) You can order online from Amazon.com at:

http://www.amazon.com

Search for this book by title or by the ISBN number:

ISBN-13: 978-1-884979-05-7
ISBN-10: 1-884979-05-x

(2) For wholesale or bookstore orders, go to Ingram Book Group

http://www.ingrampublisherservices.com/retailer/default.asp

One Ingram Blvd.
P.O. Box 3006
LaVergne, TN 37086-1986

(866) 400-5351

Retailer@ingrampublisherservices.com

_____

For all other inquiries, contact the publisher by logging onto the website and using the contact form.

Published by: Clear Springs Press, LLC
             Yelm, WA   U.S.A.
http://www.clspress.com/contact.html

Table of Contents

Foreword

The search for "alternative" or natural treatments for any disease or illness is frequently frustrated by a lack of good information. On the one hand, there may be a lack of quality, published scientific information on the potential alternatives. The potential alternatives include those from traditional medical systems such as ayurvedic medicine, chinese medicine, homeopathic medicine, herbal medicine, and recent but not fully proven discoveries. The development of the high quality double blind clinical studies on viable alternatives frequently goes unsupported or even blocked by self-serving economic and political interests. The viable alternatives, then, are regarded as "unapproved." Unapproved means untested, at least in a scientifically rigorous and politically correct manner. The potentially viable alternatives are then unavailable through traditional or orthodox channels.

This leaves a vacuum in which unscrupulous promoters can operate making unsupported and unsubstantiated claims for quick financial gain. The consumer deserves better.

I have examined several of the natural and/or alternative treatments for herpes virus infections and presented them here with scientific and medical references to the extent that they are available. I have made an effort to be objective and as unbiased as possible.

I did not discuss orthodox herpes treatments. They are well covered elsewhere. I also did not discuss social aspects or traditional management of herpes infections. They are well covered elsewhere. I also did not discuss the diagnosis of herpes infections. That too, is well covered elsewhere.

Before any treatment is obtained or chosen, a diagnosis must be obtained from a qualified health care practitioner. There are a number of other health conditions or diseases that can be confused with herpes infection symptoms.

Anyone choosing to self-treat using alternative or complementary treatments should consult a physician and obtain medical advice first.

1

This information is presented for educational purposes and is not medical advice and is not intended to serve as a treatment or cure for any disease.

Some Important Terms

Unapproved - Common sense might tell you that "unapproved" means "disapproved." This is not the case. Unapproved simply means that something has not been evaluated and, therefore, has not been approved.

Complementary medicine - This term refers to systems of health care and individual therapies that people use as adjuncts to their conventional health care.

Alternative medicine - "Alternative" medicine is every available approach to healing that does not fall within the accepted norms of conventional medicine. Most new treatments and practices are regarded as alternative until they become adopted by the mainstream practitioners.

Health freedom - Some individuals, doctors, and campaigners believe that the practice of medicine has become constrained by monopoly interests and profit to the detriment of health and freedom of choice.

Evidence based medicine - Evidence based medicine aims to apply evidence gained through the scientific method to health care practice. It seeks to quantify the risks and benefits of treatments. In principle, this looks like a good idea. It is, however, sometimes biased by politics and financial interests. Because of this, some third party payers (insurance companies, HMO's etc.) may, in some cases, use "evidence based medicine" as an excuse to deny payment for services.

Chapter 1 - Herpes Virus Types

The focus of this document is on Herpes family viruses Herpes Simplex Type I (Cold Sores), Herpes Simplex Type II (Genital Herpes), and Herpes Zoster (Shingles and Chicken Pox). There are also several additional herpes viruses. Nearly everyone is carrying one or more of these viruses in their bodies, usually in a dormant state. When one of them erupts, the result can range from annoying to very painful to life threatening.

The known types of human herpes viruses infecting humans include:

- Herpes Simplex Virus Type 1 (HHV1) - The outbreaks are often called cold sores and usually occur around the mouth but can occur on the fingers, toes and genital area as well. HSV-1 and HSV-2 are very similar. Both lie dormant in nerve cell nuclei and follow the nerve distribution to the surface of skin or organs when they erupt. About 80% of Americans have oral herpes, HSV-1. It is estimated that 10% to 20% of these individuals experience recurring outbreaks of lesions.

- Herpes Simplex Virus Type 2 (HHV2) - HSV-2 usually erupts around the genital area. Like HSV-1, HSV-2 lies dormant in nerve cell nuclei and follows the nerve distribution to the surface of skin or organs when they erupt. In 1994, it was estimated that one in five people (20%) in the United States over the age of 12 was infected with HSV-2, the virus that causes genital herpes. Since the late 1970s, the number of Americans with genital herpes infection has increased 30% and approximately one million new invections are acquired every year. It is estimated that 80-90% of those with genital herpes are unaware that they are infected.

- Varicella-Zoster Virus (Herpes Zoster) (HHV3) - Herpes zoster is also called herpes varicella, chickenpox, and herpes zoster, shingles. Herpes Zoster presents as a flu-like illness followed by blisters over the body. Like

HSV-1 and HSV-2 the virus lies dormant in the nuclei of nerve cells. When outbreaks occur, they follow the dermatome distribution of the nerves. Anyone who has had chickenpox is carrying the virus and is at risk of a shingles outbreak. It is estimated that approximately 10 to 20 percent of Americans will experience a shingles outbreak. There are approximately 500,000 cases of shingles in the United States every year.

- Epstein Barr Virus (EBV) (HHV4) - Epstein barr virus is also called glandular fever, mononucleosis, mono, and kissing disease. In babies and children, the symptoms are often so mild that they are not noticed. In teenagers and adults it causes a fever, swollen glands, aching joints, and it may cause ongoing fatigue. In the United States up to 95% of the adult population has been infected with EBV. EBV also establishes a lifelong dormant infection in some cells of the body's immune system. EBV may be associated with two rare cancers known as Burkitt's lymphoma and nasopharyngeal carcinoma.

- Cytomegalovirus (CMV) (HHV5) - This virus is present in saliva, breast milk, and other secretions. In adults, it is usually caught with no symptoms at all. Sometimes it causes the same symptoms as a mild glandular fever. HCMV infects between 50% and 80% of adults in the United States. Some individuals with symptoms experience an infectious mononucleosis like symptoms with prolonged fever, mild hepatitis, and sore throat.

- Human Herpes Virus 6 (HHV6) - There are two distinct types of HHV6, designated 6A and 6B. Type 6B causes roseola in babies between 6 months and 1 year old. By age 2, almost all babies have type 6B virus. Symptoms include a mild fever lasting for a few days, swollen glands, and a normally mild rash which appears after the fever goes. HHV-6 primary infections account for up to 20% of infant hospitalizations in the United States and are associated with more severe complications, including encephalitis, myocarditis,

4

lympadenopathy, and melosuppression. After the primary infection, latency is established in myeloid and bone marrow tissues and exists for the life time of the host. 20-25% of healthy adults in the United States test positive for HHV6. HHV6 has also been found in multiple sclerosis patients and has been implicated in several other diseases, including chronic fatigue syndrome, AIDS, temporal lobe epilepsy, and fibromyalgia.

- Human Herpes Virus 7 (HHV7) - By the age of 3, almost all children are infected with HHV7. HHV7 and is usually transmitted through saliva, and in older people, possibly semen and other secretions. Human herpes virus (HHV6) and HHV7 are ubiquitous T-lymphotropic viruses that infect most humans.

- Human Herpes Virus 8 (HHV8) - HHV8 is also known as Karposi's sarcoma herpes virus (KSHV). It is associated with HIV infections.

Outbreaks of herpes virus infections are generally associated with events and circumstances that weaken the immune system. A depressed immune system allows the viruses to multiply and spread.

The discussion of alternative treatments for herpes viruses in this text applies primarily to HSV-1, HSV-2, and Herpes Zoster. However, some may be applicable to the other herpes family viruses as well.

The current medications used for herpes have the disadvantages of being very expensive, not offering a cure, and having potentially harmful side effects.

HSV-1, HSV-2, and Herpes Zoster viral infections have several characteristics in common:

- In their dormant state they reside in the nuclei of nerve cells in the brain or spinal column.

- When they become active they multiply and follow the nerve fibers to the surface where they erupt as lesions on the skin.

- They can all have the potential of extremely serious complications leading to severe neuralgias, pain, heart disease, vision loss, organ damage, and even death.

- They are all lipid coated viruses.

- The measures discussed in this document probably affect all three viruses in a similar manner.

- They can all be transmitted to others through viruses shed from active lesions.

Chapter 2 - Natural, Alternative, and Complementary Treatments

The modalities descibed here may affect the herpes viruses and herpes virus infections in a variety of ways.

- Some may have anti-viral properties.
- Some may interfere with viral replication.
- Some may interfere with the virus' ability to infect healthy tissue.
- Some may limit inflammation.
- Some may promote the healing of lesions.
- Some may support or boost the immune system.

Some of these supplements may offer more than one useful mechanism of action.

Herpes virus outbreaks and other infections occur when the immune system is compromised or weakened. The immune system can be compromised by stress, nutritional deficiencies, suboptimum nutrition, and age.

Stress is one of the most common and powerful immune system suppressors. Stress causes hormonal changes which directly inhibit the function of the immune system. Stress management is extremely important for infection prevention and treatment. Methods of dealing with stress are beyond the scope of this book.

Nutritional deficiencies produce overt symptoms such as goiter from iodine deficiency, scurvy from vitamin C deficiency, etc. Suboptimum nutrition, on the other hand, means that the classical overt symptoms of deficiencies may not be present, but supplementation of key nutrients may produce greater health, more energy, or improved immune system function.

Age can also be a factor in immune system efficiency but seems to be less of factor than stress or poor nutrition.

In addition to improving immune function by optimum nutrition and stress management, there are several substances which specifically boost immune function. These include Thymic Protein A, Beta Glucan, Lactoferrin, and an over the counter drug called Cimetadine.

The next section provides a brief summary of the nutritional factors and alternative treatments for herpes virus infections and possibly some related viral infections. It is recommended that you read the full chapter on each modality. The references on each modality are included at the end of the book and listed by chapter.

Chapter 3 - The Effect of Supplements on Herpes Virus Infections

One may be able to reduce the frequency and duration of herpes outbreaks through nutritional measures. There are some nutrients that support the function of the immune system and pose no risk of adverse effects. The first step is to ensure that these nutrients are supplemented to optimum levels. This includes vitamin A, vitamin C, zinc, selenium, and vitamin E. A general multiple vitamin and multiple mineral supplement is also suggested.

The next step is to supplement those nutrients that have either direct anti-viral properties or in some other way support the body's ability to resist the viral agents. The first choices here are coconut oil and lactoferrin. Both are standard foodstuffs with no known adverse effects when consumed in moderate amounts. Coconut oil in the recommended dosage has anti-viral properties and lactoferrin has both anti-viral effects and immune modulating properties. Omega-3 oils may not have much direct effect on herpes virus outbreaks, but have multiple health benefits and may help reduce the severity of outbreaks through anti-inflammatory properties.

Beta Glucan and thymic protein A both have immune system boosting properties and have no known adverse effects. The role that they may or not play in reducing the frequency and duration of herpes outbreaks is untested, but improving the immune systems' function improves the body's abililty to resist infections in general.

The amino acid Lysine when combined with restriction of the amino acid Arginine has been shown to reduce the replication of herpes viruses. This measure has been demonstrated to reduce the frequency and duration of outbreaks.

With a little luck and attention to stress reduction, these measures may be helpful in reducing the frequency and duration of herpes outbreaks. If these alone are insufficient, consider using one of these additional treatments.

Additional candidates for natural supplements with herpes anti-viral effects include green tea, resveratrol, olive leaf extract, propolis, garlic, proteolytic enzymes, and indole-3 carbinol. These substances have all demonstrated anti-viral properties against the herpes viruses in the laboratory. None of them have been tested in humans.

BHT appears to be one of the singular most effective of the alternative anti-viral supplements for herpes viruses. This is based mostly on anecdotal and unverified information. Its adverse effects appear to be minimal, or possibly non-existent, when used in the dosages outlined and with the precautions noted. However, it lacks formal studies in humans. Its anti-viral properties have been studied in the laboratory and in animals. This paragraph is not intended to be taken as medical advice and is not intended as a recommendation to use this supplement. While this supplement is sold without a prescription, one should consult with their physician and pharmacist before using it as a treatment for any illness or disease.

Cimetadine is an over the counter medication that has not been approved for treating herpes infections. Nevertheless, it has been demonstrated to up-regulate the immune sustem and has had limited and successful clinical trials in humans. It was successful in reducing the severity and duration of outbreaks of herpes simplex and herpes zoster infections. While this medication is sold without a prescription, one should consult with their physician and pharmacist before using it as a treatment for any illness or disease.

Chapter 4 - Nutritional Factors that Boost the Immune System

All diseases are prevented, suppressed, or cured by the human immune system. Even antibiotics and anti-viral medications only succeed in suppressing the growth of pathogens or in reducing their populations. Without the immune system these treatments would not be successful. It is, therefore, imperative that we do everything possible to assist our immune system to do what it is designed to do.

Immune system support nutrients include vitamin A, vitamin C, vitamin E, zinc, and selenium. Supplements that have the additional effect of boosting or stimulating the immune system include Thymic Protein A, Beta Glucan, and Lactoferrin. The over the counter drug, cimetadine, also has the effect of up-regulating the immune system.

The typical dosage of these supplements is as follows:

Vitamin A - (For adults only) 25,000 to 50,000 IU per day for one to two weeks, then reduce the dosage to 10,000 IU per day or 25,000 IU every other day. For children or women who are pregnant or who may become pregnant it may be advisable to stick to the RDA guidelines. Use natural vitamin A rather than synthetic forms. (Read the full chapter on vitamin A.)

Vitamin C - 2,000 to 5,000 mg per day in five divided doses. (Read the full chapter on vitamin C.)

Vitamin E - 200 to 400 IU per day in the form of natural vitamin E with mixed tocopherols.

Zinc - 25 mg twice per day while fighting an outbreak or during healing and 25 mg per day for maintenance. (Read the full chapter on zinc.)

Selenium - 200 mcg per day.

For some individuals, the use of these immune boosting supplements may be sufficient to keep outbreaks in check. When they are insufficient on their own, the addition of anti-viral agents should be considered.

Lactoferrin - Lactoferrin is a protein that is synthesized in the human body and is found in all bodily secretions and in the mucosa of all bodily orifices. It has both immune enhancing and imune modulatory effects and direct anti-microbial properties. Lactoferrin is beneficial in resisting HSV-1 and HSV-2 including acyclovir resistant strains. A typical daily dose is 200 to 400 mg per day during an outbreak. It can also be used for maintenance and outbreak suppression. Because lactoferrin is a food derived from milk, there is no known harm in using larger doses. The only conceivable contraindication would be in individuals with milk allergies. While there is evidence to suggest that lactoferrin may be beneficial in treating and preventing herpes outbreaks, there is induffient data to establish it as a treatment or cure on its own. (Read the full chapter on Lactoferrin.)

Beta 1,3 Glucan - Beta 1,3 Glucan is a polysaccharide derived from the cell wall of baker's yeast, oat and barley fiber, and many medicinal mushrooms, such as Reishi, Shiitake, and Maitake. Studies have shown that beta 1,3 glucan activates macrophages and neutrophils. For enhancing immune function, an effective amount has not yet been determined. Manufacturers of beta glucan products usually recommend between 50 and 1,000 mg daily.

Thymic Protein A - Thymic Protein A stimulates the immune system by supporting thymus function. Thymus activity diminishes with age, stress, disease. and suboptimum nutrition. Thymic Protein A is a protein that has been formulated for effective absorption through the sublingual mucosa. Administration is by placing a packet of powder under the tongue and holding it there where it is absorbed directly into the blood stream. A maintenance or preventive dose would be one packet every other day. For an active outbreak, three packets per day is a good dose (based on the manufacturer's suggestions). The effect of thymic protein A is a non-specific stimulation of the immune system. Its precise impact on herpes infections has not been studied. (Read the full chapter on thymic protein A.)

Cimetadine - Cimetadine is sold as an over the counter drug for treating heartburn. It is not approved for the treatment of herpes infections. However, it has been clinically tested for HSV-2 and HZV infections and found effective. It is sometimes prescribed for this application by both alternative and traditional physicians. Cimetadine is not an anti-viral drug. Rather, it up-regulates the immune system to make the body more resistant to all types of infections. The dosage used in the clinical trials on cimetadine and herpes was <u>200 mg three times daily and 400 mg at night</u>. If cimetidine is used, it should be initiated as soon as the first symptoms of a herpes outbreak manifest and should be continued until the lesion disappears. It would not be prudent for one to take cimetidine continuously for prevention. <u>Consult your pharmacist or physician before using Cimetadine as a treatment for herpes or any other disease. Pay particular attention to the package insert for drug interactions and side effects.</u> (Read the full chapter on cimetadine.)

Chapter 5 - Nutritional Substances with Anti-Viral Properties

Coconut Oil - Take <u>4 tablespoons per day (minimum)</u> as food. Try replacing other oils, butter, etc. with coconut oil rather than taking it as a separate supplement. Coconut oil contains lauric acid which solubilizes the lipid coat of the herpes viruses making them more vulnerable to the human immune system. Coconut oil is a food and has no adverse effects when used as a food. (Read the full chapter on coconut oil.)

BHT - BHT also solubilizes the lipid coat of the virus and should act very synergistically with coconut oil in particular and other measures in general. Read the entire section on BHT and be familiar with the listed precautions. The available references suggest that <u>dosages should start small, about 250 mg per day for 2-3 days to see if there is any allergic sensitivity to it. Then increase the dosage in increments up to 1000 mg per day.</u> Some physicians recommend using as high as 3000 mg during an outbreak. Some individuals have reported side effects at this dosage. If you have liver disease, or you are using more than 1000 mg per day, or you are using it long term as a preventive, you should have your liver enzymes monitored. If liver enzymes become elevated, you should reduce the dose or discontinue BHT consumption.

BHT has not been formally researched as a treatment of herpes infections in humans. It has demonstrated anti-viral effects in vitro and in animals. It has been used as a life extension anti-oxidant and an off label anti-viral medication by a significant and unknown number of individuals. The anecdotal information about BHT suggests that it is generally effective in suppressing herpes outbreaks and generally safe within the precautions noted. BHT is approved by the FDA as a food preservative. <u>If you choose to use BHT as a herpes treatment, consult your physician first. Consult your pharmacist to assess the possibility of drug interactions with any medications that you may be using.</u> (Read the full chapter on BHT.)

Again, please note that BHT has not been tested in humans and probably never will be. BHT is inexpensive and unpatentable. If its effectiveness and safety were formally documented, it might displace some very expensive anti-viral medications. No private company would profit from the expense of doing such research. Public funding for such projects is subject to political processes.

Coconut oil and BHT suppress herpes viruses by the same mechanism of action. It is therefore likely that using the two together would increase their overall effectiveness. There are some products on the market that consist of BHT dissolved in coconut oil. These products are intended for topical application.

Lysine - Lysine is an essential amino acid. It has no direct anti-viral properties but has been demonstrated to reduce the replication of herpes viruses when there is also a shortage of the essential amino acid arginine. This does not kill the virus but does slow it down. To be effective, arginine intake must also be restricted. Given that arginine is an essential amino acid, long term restriction is not a good idea. Some of the other measures are apparently more effective than lysine supplementation and arginine restriction. It could be used as an adjunct to other measures during outbreaks if needed. The dosage of lysine usually recommended is 1,000 - 3,000 mg per day. (Read the full chapter on lysine.)

Garlic - Garlic is a common food and has been proven to have broad spectrum germicidal properties. Some sources suggest that an appropriate garlic dosage during an outbreak is two 1000-mg capsules two times daily or four 500 mg capsules two times daily. Other than the associated odor and possible belching, garlic is considered safe and without adverse effects. This is a general health measure as well as a specific therapeutic intervention. The use of garlic in treating herpes outbreaks has not been sufficiently documented to make any statements about its effectiveness. (Read the full garlic chapter.)

Propolis - Propolis is a material found in bee hives and is known to have broad spectrum germicidal properties. The only contraindication is for individuals who have a possible allergy to it. Some sources suggest a dosage of one to four propolis capsules daily (400 mg). Propolis is not recommended for individuals with an allergy to tree resin or bee stings. The use of propolis in treating herpes outbreaks is not sufficiently documented to make any statements about its effectiveness in humans. (Read the full chapter on propolis.)

Proteolytic Enzymes - Proteolytic Enzymes have non specific immune enhancing and anti-inflammatory properties. To have an effect, they must be taken on an empty stomach between meals, one hour before eating and two or more hours after eating. There are several different proteolytic enzymes and combinations of enzymes on the market in varying strengths. If you use them follow the label instructions. You may have to experiment with the dosage to get the desired effect. There is some documentation to support this application for herpes, but not enough to claim that it is generally effective. (Read the full chapter on proteolytic enzymes.)

Indole-3-Carbinol (I3C) - Indole-3-Carbinol (I3C) is a compound extracted from cruciferous vegetables. It has broad health benefits and has been shown to have specific anti-viral activity against HSV-1 and HSV-2 in laboratory experiments. Human experiments have not yet been done. I3C is broken down into several derivative products in the digestive tract. The anti-viral properties of these derivative products are not as well known. One derivative, DIM, has demonstrated several health benefits, but its effect on viruses is not clearly documented.

Resveratrol - Resveratrol is a compound found in red grapes, peanuts, and a few other plants. Resveratrol has many health benefits and has demonstrated broad anti-viral properties in laboratory studies. It is somewhat unclear whether or not it has the same anti-viral effects in humans when administered orally. Nevertheless, it deserves to be included in one's supplement regimen because of its numerous other health benefits.

Green Tea - Green tea has been demonstrated to have some anti-viral properties in the laboratory. There have been some anecdotal reports of individuals keeping herpes outbreaks suppressed with green tea and resveratrol only. There are some health concerns about the aluminum and fluoride content of tea, including green tea. For this reason, aluminum and fluoride free extracts are favored over the tea infusion. No anti-viral dose of green tea has been established.

Olive Leaf Extract - Research has demonstrated that olive leaf extract has antimicrobial properties that affect viruses, bacteria, fungus, yeast, and protozoa. The list specifically includes the herpes viruses. However, all of the testing was in the laboratory, not in human trials. A dosage for treating humans with olive leaf extract has not been determined.

Omega-3 Fatty Acids - Omega-3 fatty acids have general anti-inflammatory effects, may strengthen cell walls to help resist viral invasion and may have a degree of direct anti-viral properties. An optimum dose is <u>2,000 mg of EPA and 1,000 mg of DHA per day</u>.

Chapter 6 - Vitamin A

Vitamin A is commonly known as the anti-infective vitamin, because it is required for normal functioning of the immune system. (9) Vitamin A plays several rolls in herpes virus outbreaks. It is a factor in skin and mucous membrane integrity, in the healing of lesions, and in the integrity and efficiency of the immune system.

In one study, 178 HIV-positive women with genital herpes were monitored for vitamin A levels and cervical HSV shedding. Increased viral shedding was associated with decreased vitamin A. (1)

Other experimental studies have documented vitamin A's effectiveness against other herpes family viruses. The strong anti-proliferative activity exerted by retinoids (vitamin A derivatives) indicates these compounds may be useful tools in the management of EBV–related disorders in immuno-suppressed patients. (2)

In another controlled, double-blind study, the effects of 10 to 12 years of beta-carotene supplementation on natural killer (NK) cell activity were evaluated. Elderly men who took supplements of beta-carotene had significantly greater NK cell activity than the control group receiving placebo. Beta-carotene is a precursor to vitamin A and can be assumed to have increased the level of active vitamin A in the test subjects. (3)

Most research shows that vitamin A is beneficial to the immune system and mucus membranes. This is especially true in the elderly and those in developing countries where deficiencies are common. (5, 6) Individuals who do not have deficiencies tend not to show immune system enhancement from vitamin A alone.

There is, however, evidence that combinations of supplements can be far more effective than a single supplement. In two studies, a significant increase in immune cell numbers was observed in the group that received a combination of vitamin A, vitamin C, and vitamin E. The patients in this study were elderly. (7, 8)

Vitamin A plays a central role in the development and differentiation of white blood cells, such as lymphocytes, which play critical roles in the immune response. Activation of T-lymphocytes, the major regulatory cells of the immune system, appears to require vitamin A. *(11)*

It is quite clear that a vitamin A deficiency can increase your vulnerability to infection, but overdosing can be harmful. Getting less than the government recommendation of 5,000 International Units of vitamin A can:

- Reduce the size of your thymus gland
- Reduce the number of lymphocytes that you have
- Reduce the production of antibodies to fight infections
- Reduce the capacity of the respiratory tract to expel pathogens

Vitamin A Dosage

Vitamin supplements may contain one or more of retinyl acetate and retinyl palmitate and beta carotene. Rarely are doses higher than 5,000 IU of vitamin A exceeded in these formulas. The beta carotene content does not count toward the vitamin A dosage from a toxicological standpoint. Many take beta-carotene for vitamin A supplements for this reason. Vitamin A is also available in the form of cod liver oil.

The current recommended dietary allowances (RDA) for vitamin A by the Food and Nutrition Board of the U.S. National Academy of Sciences are:

- Infants up to 1 year old - 1,250 IU per day
- Children 1 through 3 years old - 1,333 IU per day
- Children 4 through 6 years old - 1,667 IU per day
- Children 7 through 10 years old - 2,333 IU per day
- Males 11 years and older - 3,333 IU per day
- Females 11 years and older - 3,333 IU per day
- Pregnant/Lactating 1st 6 months - 4,333 IU per day
- Pregnant/Lactating 2nd 6 months - 4,000 IU per day

One IU or one USP unit equals 0.30 micrograms of all-trans retinol, 0.344 micrograms of retinyl acetate or 0.55 micrograms of retinyl palmitate. *(12)*

Remember that the RDA is the dose that is believed to prevent the symptoms of deficiency disease. The dosage that provides optimum health and disease resistance is likely higher than the RDA. Unfortunately, there is no research data showing what optimum levels are. The optimum level for different individuals is likely to vary because of different genetics and metabolic needs. The fact that vitamin A can be toxic means that one must be cautious about overdosing.

Vitamin A and Birth Defects

Since a 1995 report from the *New England Journal of Medicine,* there has been some concern that pregnant women taking too much vitamin A could be increasing their risk of birth defects. *(13)* The upper limit referenced is 10,000 IU per day.

A more recent report studied several hundred women exposed to 10,000–300,000 IU (median exposure of 50,000 IU) per day. *(14)* Three major malformations occurred in this study. However, no congenital malformations happened in any of the 120 infants exposed to maternal intakes of vitamin A that exceeded 50,000 IU per day. The high-exposure group had a 50% decreased risk for malformations compared with infants not exposed to vitamin A. The authors noted that some previous studies found no link between vitamin A and birth defects, and argued the studies that did find such a link suffered from various weaknesses.

A closer look at this study reveals a 32% higher than expected risk of birth defects in infants exposed to 10,000–40,000 IU of vitamin A per day, but a 37% decreased risk for those exposed to even higher levels. This suggests that defects from both "higher" and "lower" risks may have been due to chance.

Excessive dietary intake of vitamin A has been associated with birth defects in humans in fewer than 20 reported cases over the past 30 years. *(15, 16)* Presently, the level at which vitamin A supplementation may cause birth defects is not known, though combined human and animal data suggest that 30,000 IU per day should be considered safe. *(17)* Women who are or who could become pregnant should consult with a doctor before supplementing with more than 10,000 IU per day.

Vitamin A Toxicity and Over dosage

The potential for greatest harm from vitamin A toxicity is first to the unborn and second to young children. Research has shown that both excess and deficiency can be harmful. More research is needed to clarify what the boundaries in dosage are. For now, it may be wise to stick to the RDA numbers if pregnant, nursing, or very young.

Carotenoids, such as beta-carotene, are not vitamin A. Rather, they are pro-vitamin A. They must be converted to vitamin A in the liver. They help regulate three types of immune cells: T and B lymphocytes, natural killer cells, and macrophages.

There is some evidence that vitamin A from natural sources may be less toxic than vitamin A from synthetic sources. Fat-soluble vitamin A naturally found in foods like cod liver oil, liver, and butterfat may be safe at up to ten times the doses of water-soluble, solidified, and emulsified vitamin A found in some supplements that produce toxicity. *(18)*

Acute toxicity generally occurs at doses of 25,000 IU/kg, with chronic toxicity occurring at 4,000 IU/kg daily for 6-15 months. *(19)* Liver toxicities can occur at levels as low as 15,000 IU per day to 1.4 million IU per day, with an average daily toxic dose of 120,000 IU per day. In people with renal failure 4000 IU can cause substantial damage.

In chronic cases of hypervitaminosis A, hair loss, drying of the mucous membranes, fever, insomnia, fatigue, weight loss, bone fractures, anemia, and diarrhea can all be evident on top of the symptoms associated with less serious toxicity. *(20)*

Most of the reported cases of vitamin A toxicity and over dosage have been from arctic explorers who consumed the livers of polar animals, polar bears, dogs, and seals in particular. There have been very few reports of fatalities from high doses of vitamin A.

The remedy for an overdose of vitamin A is to stop taking vitamin A supplements or eating polar bear livers until the symptoms subside.

Vitamin A Summary

Vitamin A is an important supplement for preventing and relieving herpes outbreaks. Its effectiveness is greatest when combined with the other vitamins and minerals that also support immune system function.

Chapter 7 - Vitamin C - The Most Essential Nutrient

Vitamin C is one of the most researched, studied, and written about substances in scientific and medical literature. There are over 24,000 citations on vitamin C listed in the scientific and medical literature.

Ascorbic Acid (Vitamin C) is a vitamin only because it is a nutrient essential for life that is not manufactured in the body and must be obtained from outside sources. Every living thing on this planet, except primates (including man), some bats, and guinea pigs, produce their own Vitamin C internally, do not require it in their diet, and do not suffer from a host of diseases and maladies caused by Vitamin C deficiencies.

Vitamin C is manufactured internally from glucose by a four-step process, each requiring a specific enzyme. Humans have the first three enzymes but the fourth is damaged and non functional apparently from a genetic mutation that occurred in our distant ancestors. It seems that we really have a species-wide genetic disease. Perhaps fixing this genetic defect should be a primary goal for the genetic engineers of this century.

Vitamin C and Herpes

Vitamin C is necessary in maintaining immune status. Vitamin C strengthens white blood cell function and boosts interferon levels. Vitamin C is a free radical scavenger and protects tissues from oxidative stress. *(1)*

In one clinical trial, a water-soluble bioflavonoid/ascorbic acid complex (600 to 1000 milligrams [mg] of bioflavonoids and 600 to 1000 mg of ascorbic acid taken three to five times daily) was shown to be effective in the reduction of recurrent HSV1, reducing blisters, and preventing disruption of vesicular membranes. Remission of symptoms was observed in 4 days. *(2)*

In another study on the topical treatment of recurrent mucocutaneous herpes, a pharmaceutical ascorbic acid formulation demonstrated the anti-viral effects of vitamin C. A cotton pad soaked in the solution was firmly pressed on the lesion for 2 minutes three times for one day only. The treatment resulted in markedly reduced symptoms and fewer days of scab formation. *(3)*

What Vitamin C Does for Us

What does vitamin C do for us? There is not one body process and not one disease or syndrome that is not influenced by vitamin C.

Vitamin C is an antioxidant acting to reduce oxidative stress. *(4)* It is also an enzyme cofactor for the biosynthesis of numerous substances that are essential for human health. There are at least eight enzymes for which vitamin C acts as an electron donor. *(5)*

Essential functions that require vitamin C include:

- Collagen Synthesis *(6 - 9)*

- Carnitine Synthesis and ATP function for energy generation *(10, 11)*

- Stabilizes peptide hormones *(14,15)*

- Enhanced Immune Function *(20)*

- Synthesis of the neurotransmitters norepinephrine and dopamine *(12, 13)*

Vitamin C Enhances Immune Function

Vitamin C has been found to inhibit viral infectivity by inactivating viruses and by affecting viral replication. Additionally, vitamin C promotes immunological functions, such as phagocytosis, chemotaxis, and neutrophil adhesion, and acts as a powerful antioxidant thereby alleviating oxidative stress and the associated inflammation by viral infection. Ascorbate is also involved in the synthesis of crucial immune system molecules, such as cytokines, antibodies, and interferon. *(20)*

Vitamin C and Collagen Synthesis

Collagen is the foundation of all connective tissue, literally everything that holds the body together. Scurvy is the result of deterioration of the blood vessels resulting in hemorrhage, bleeding gums, bruising, loose teeth, tendency of bones to fracture, etc. Maladies affecting tendons, ligaments, skin, bone, teeth, cartilage, heart valves, intervertebral discs, cornea, and eye lens also result from vitamin C deficiency. There is a long continuum between scurvy and optimum tissue integrity. *(6 - 9)*

How Much Vitamin C do We Need?

The North American Dietary Reference Intake recommends 90 mg per day and no more than 2 grams per day. *(21)* Other related species sharing the same inability to produce vitamin C and requiring exogenous vitamin C consume 20 to 80 times this reference intake. *(22, 23)*

Irwin Stone and Linus Pauling calculated that the optimum daily requirement of vitamin C is around 2,300 milligrams for a human requiring 2,500 kcal a day. This estimate is based on the diet of our primate cousins (similar to what our distant ancestors are likely to have consumed when the gene mutated). *(21 - 23)*

In the 1960s Linus Pauling began actively promoting vitamin C as a means to greatly improve human health and resistance to disease. His book *How to Live Longer and Feel Better* was a bestseller and advocated taking more than 10,000 milligrams per day orally, thus approaching the amounts released by the liver directly into the circulation in other mammals. A goat, for example, will manufacture more than 13,000 mg of vitamin C per day in normal health and as much as 100,000 mg daily when faced with life-threatening disease, trauma, or stress. *(24)*

Vitamin C Orthomolecular Therapy

Orthomolecular therapy or mega dose therapy is the use of either oral or intravenous doses of vitamin C that are much larger than the daily recommended intake. A number of scientists and physicians have advocated this approach. One doctor who championed high dose vitamin C was Frederich Klenner, M.D. He published extensively on the successful treatment of polio and many other infectious diseases including herpes infections. Dr. Klenner's protocols used very large dosages often administered by intramuscular injection and intravenously. He reported generally successful outcomes of his treatments. *(26)*

Doses in the range of 10 to over 200 grams per day have been used. One rationale for higher doses is that primates in their native environment consume 50 to 80 times as much vitamin C as the official reference intake for humans. *(27, 28)*

Other Therapeutic Uses

In 1990, the <u>Proceedings of National Academy of Sciences</u> published a study showing that non toxic doses of vitamin C suppress HIV replication *in vitro*. *(29)* To date, no large scale clinical trials have been done to exploit this potential.

Numerous studies have investigated the use of vitamin C as a cancer treatment or cancer adjunctive treatment. In January 2007 the US <u>Food and Drug Administration</u> approved a Phase I toxicity trial to determine the safe dosage of intravenous vitamin C as a possible cancer treatment. *(30)*

Vitamin C has demonstrated the ability to reduce lead levels in the blood. 1000 mg of vitamin C per day reduced the blood lead levels by 81% while lower doses were ineffective.
(32, 31)

Vitamin C Precautions and Side Effects

Some of the factors that someone taking vitamin C should be aware of include:

- Vitamin C increases iron absorption and decreases copper absorption
- Vitamin C can react with some medications

26

- The acid form of vitamin C may aggravate stomach ulcers
- Large doses of Vitamin C is contraindicated with certain blood diseases including sickle-cell anemia, hemochromatosis, and thalassemia
- Large doses of the acid form of Vitamin C can cause diarrhea

Vitamin C has been reported to cause kidney stones through the formation of oxalic acid. While this claim is often quoted by critics of vitamin C therapy, the evidence indicates this claim is false. *(33)* Vitamin C has been reported to cause thickening of the coronary arteries. The evidence indicates that this claim is false. *(34)* Vitamin C has been reported to increase the risk of cancer under some circumstances. The evidence indicates that this claim is false. *(35)* It has been reported that too much vitamin C can cause genetic damage. The evidence indicates that this claim is false. *(36)*

Chapter 8 - Zinc

Zinc is an essential element, necessary for sustaining life. Zinc is essential as an enzyme activating cofactor in over 300 of the body's critical functions, including the production of T-lymphocytes. It is estimated that 3,000 of the hundreds of thousands of proteins in the human body contain zinc. In addition, there are over a dozen types of cells in the human body that secrete zinc ions that act as messengers or signals. The roles of these secreted zinc signals in medicine and health are now being actively studied. Zinc ions are now considered neurotransmitters. Cells in the salivary gland, prostate, immune system, and intestine use zinc signaling. *(1)* A zinc deficiency is a health disaster.

Zinc Deficiency

A deficiency of zinc has been demonstrated to have the following effects on the human body: *(2, 3)*

- Shrinks the size of the thymus gland
- Reduces the number of lymphocytes
- Slows the production of lymphocytes
- Impairs the function of lymphocytes and macrophages
- Decreases the antibody response
- Prevents wounds from healing properly
- Slows growth and development
- Delays sexual maturation
- Causes characteristic skin rashes
- Causes chronic and severe diarrhea
- Causes diminished appetite
- Causes impaired taste sensation
- Causes night blindness
- Causes swelling and clouding of the corneas
- Causes behavioral disturbances

Data from the Third National Health and Nutrition Examination Survey (NHANES III) suggest that "mild [zinc] deficiency is . . . common in the US." *(40)*

Zinc and Immune Function

The immune system is adversely affected by even slight zinc deficiency and seriously depressed by severe zinc deficiency. *(4)* When zinc supplements are given to individuals with low zinc levels, the numbers of T-cell lymphocytes circulating in the blood increase and the ability of lymphocytes to fight infection improves. *(5)* Zinc deficient individuals are known to experience increased susceptibility to a variety of infectious agents. Zinc is necessary for proper T cell and natural killer cell function and proper lymphocyte activity. Zinc is directly involved in antibody production to help fight infection. *(6)*

Zinc and Herpes

There is evidence that Zinc may be an effective modality for treating both Herpes type I and Herpes type II. Zinc has been used both as oral therapy and externally as a topical preparation. Taken internally, zinc would be beneficial by boosting immune function, promoting more rapid healing of lesions, and possibly anti-viral effects. Topically, zinc ions are noted to kill viruses on contact.

Zinc is a specific activator of T-cells, T-cell division, and other immune cellular functions. Zinc also functions as an antioxidant and stabilizes membranes against the oxidative damage by increasing the levels of catalase, superoxide dismutase, and glutathione-S-transferase. Zinc-deficient patients display reduced resistance to infection. *(8)*

In a double-blind, placebo-controlled, randomized clinical trial that evaluated the effect of a zinc oxide/glycine cream on facial herpes in 46 patients, treatment reduced or shortened the duration of cold sore lesions when applied within 24 hours of onset of symptoms. The cream also reduced the severity of symptoms. *(9)*

Selenium may help suppress the reactivation of herpes viruses by increasing immunity. A number of studies have shown that the combination of zinc and selenium enhances immunity in the elderly. A study published in Lancet found that seniors taking modest doses of a multivitamin/multimineral supplement containing zinc and selenium showed a general reduction in infection and required antibiotics for significantly fewer days annually. *(10)*

Another randomized, placebo-controlled, double-blind study found that seniors taking zinc and selenium together had significantly fewer infections, but that vitamin supplementation alone did not have a major effect. The zinc and selenium supplement cut the number of infections by nearly two-thirds, compared to placebo. *(11)*

For topical application, zinc oxide ointment is recommended for men but not women. Drying agents should not be used in the vaginal area. Use a disposable glove or cotton swab to apply medication to HHV3, HSV-1 and HSV-2 to prevent spread of the infection. Another topical form is zinc gluconate. Zinc lozenges are frequently used with sore throats for their antimicrobial effects. They can also be used with cold sores in cases where the lozenges can come in contact with the lesions. *(12 - 17)*

An article that discusses the topical application of zinc for various types of herpes lesions can be found at:

http://george-eby-research.com/html/herpes.html

Zinc Requirements Daily Reference Intakes

The daily reference intakes of zinc by age are: *(18)*

Infants

0 - 6 months   2 (mg/day)
7 - 12 months 3 (mg/day)

Children

1 - 3 years   3 (mg/day)
4 - 8 years   5 (mg/day)

Pregnancy

< 18 years   13 (mg/day)
19-30 years   11(mg/day)
31-50 years   11(mg/day)

Lactation

< 18 years   14(mg/day)
19-30 years   12(mg/day)
31-50 years   12(mg/day)

Males

9 - 13 years   8 (mg/day)
14 - 18 years 11(mg/day)
19 - 30 years 11(mg/day)
31 - 50 years 11(mg/day)
51 - 70 years 11(mg/day)
> 70 years   11(mg/day)

Females

9 - 13 years   8 (mg/day)
14 - 18 years 9 (mg/day)
19 - 30 years 8 (mg/day)
31 - 50 years 8 (mg/day)
51 - 70 years 8 (mg/day)
> 70 years   8 (mg/day

Zinc Toxicity

While a zinc deficiency is a health disaster, once the body's needs have been met, more is not better.

If you take too much zinc, you may experience zinc toxicity, which may result in abdominal cramping, diarrhea, and vomiting.

Excessive zinc intake will eventually affect the balance and proper ratios to numerous other important nutrients that may include iron, calcium, selenium, nickel, phosphorus, copper, as well as Vitamin A, B1, C, and others.

Long term overdosing on zinc may also cause, or contribute to gastrointestinal problems, hair loss, anemia, loss of libido, impotence, prostatitis, ovarian cysts, menstrual problems, depressed immune functions, muscle spasms, sciatica, renal tubular necrosis, interstitial nephritis, dizziness, and vomiting among others.

Zinc toxicity may also (in doses > 80 mg/day) decrease levels of HDL-cholesterol and white blood cells. Impaired cholesterol metabolism may also result from excess intake of zinc supplements.

The upper limit of safety for zinc established by the Food and Nutrition Board of the Institute of Medicine is 40 milligrams daily for adults.

The Zinc Tolerable Upper Intake Levels for different life stages are: *(18)*

Infants	Children	Males, Females
0-6 months	1-3 years	9-13 years
4 (mg/day)	7 (mg/day)	23 (mg/day)
7-12 months	4-8 years	14-18 years
5 (mg/day)	12 (mg/day)	34 (mg/day)
		19-70 years
Pregnancy	Lactation	40 (mg/day)
< 18 years	< 18 years	
34 (mg/day)	34 (mg/day)	> 70 years
		40 (mg/day)
19-50 years	19-50 years	
40 (mg/day)	40 (mg/day)	

Zinc Deficiency Test

Several methods have been used to assess zinc status. They include measuring the zinc content in plasma, serum, leukocyte, muscle, urine, hair, and sweat. Plasma and serum zinc content has been shown to vary widely and is influenced by a number of variables. Muscle, leukocyte, and sweat measurements are regarded as more accurate. Hair analysis can be unreliable because zinc status affects hair growth as well as mineral deposition in hair. Interestingly, the taste test has proven to be an accurate, inexpensive and readily accessible test. *(19 - 27)*

The zinc taste test is based on the knowledge that taste and smell are dependent upon the presence of sufficient zinc in the body. Thus, if zinc is deficient then taste sensation will be diminished. A standard test solution of zinc sulphate is used for tasting. The response is then compared with defined standards and the zinc status is thus estimated.

This simple, non-toxic test uses a test solution of zinc sulphate in purified water, at a concentration of 1gm/liter. The solution should be left at room temperature for about two hours before carrying out the test. To do the test, one takes approximately 5-10ml of the standard solution and holds it in the mouth exactly ten seconds. It is essential that neither food nor drink be taken for approximately one hour before the test. *(28)*

The defined standards are:

- **Grade one response:** no specific taste sensation: tastes like plain water. This indicates a major deficiency of zinc requiring supplementation to correct.

- **Grade two response:** no immediate taste is noticed, but within the ten seconds of the test, a 'dry' or 'metallic' taste is experienced. This indicates a moderate deficiency requiring supplementation to correct.

- **Grade three response:** an immediate slight taste is noted, which increases with time over the ten second period. This indicates a deficiency of minor degree requiring supplementation to correct.

- **Grade four response:** an immediate, strong, and unpleasant taste is experienced. This indicates that no zinc deficiency exists. No supplementation is required but a maintenance dose of the DRI (daily recommended intake) per day may prevent deficiencies from developing in the future.

Standardized zinc taste test solutions are commercially available and can usually be found from an internet search. Your local compounding pharmacist could also mix a batch for you.

Zinc Precautions and Side Effects

- Zinc intake in excess of 300 mg per day has been reported to impair immune function. *(29)*

- Some people report that taking zinc supplements on an empty stomach causes stomach ache, nausea, mouth irritation, and a bad taste.

- In topical form, zinc has no known side effects when used as recommended.

- Zinc nasal sprays should be avoided. There have been reports of long lasting or permanent loss of smell from using nasal sprays. *(30)*

- Zinc inhibits copper absorption. Copper intake should be increased if zinc supplementation continues for more than a few days. Evidence suggests that no more than w mg of copper per day is needed to prevent zinc induced copper deficiency. Zinc induced copper deficiency has been reported to cause reversible anemia and suppression of bone marrow. *(31)*

- Zinc competes for absorption with copper, iron, calcium, and magnesium. A multimineral supplement will help prevent mineral imbalances that can result from taking high amounts of zinc for extended periods of time. *(32 - 35)*

- N-acetyl cysteine (NAC) acts as a chelating agent and may increase urinary excretion of zinc. Long-term users of NAC may consider adding supplements of zinc and copper. *(36)*

- Some medications increase the need for zinc. The absorption of some antibiotics is impaired by zinc supplements. Consult with your pharmacist or physician when taking zinc supplements with medication.

Chapter 9 - Lactoferrin

Lactoferrin is a minor glycoprotein component of whey. It belongs to the iron transporter or transferrin family of glycoproteins. Lactoferrin is also found in exocrine secretions from mammals and is released from neutrophil granules during inflammation. The lactoferrin concentration in bovine (cows) milk is only 0.5% to 1.0% while human breast milk can contain as much as 15% lactoferrin.

Lactoferrin plays several important roles in human biology. First, Lactoferrin is believed to play a role in the uptake and absorption of iron through the intestinal mucosa. It may be the primary or sole source of iron for breast fed infants. Second, Lactoferrin appears to have anti-bacterial, anti-viral, anti-fungal, anti-inflammatory, antioxidant, and immunomodulatory activities.

Immune Support

Lactoferrin is a first line immune defense in the human body. Lactoferrin is found throughout the human body and occurs in all secretions that bathe mucous membranes such as saliva, tears, bronchial and nasal secretions, hepatic bile, pancreatic fluids, and is an essential factor in the immune response. Lactoferrin is concentrated in oral cavities where it kills or greatly suppresses pathogens. Specific receptors for lactoferrin are found on many key immune cells such as lymphocytes, monocytes and macrophages. It also up-regulates natural killer (NK) cell activity.

Research using animal models has found the ingestion of lactoferrin to have direct protective effects on the regulation and modulation of the immune system. Several studies have shown that lactoferrin significantly increased the survival rate in animals suffering from septic shock. *(1, 2)* Additional studies involving humans demonstrated that lactoferrin augments the immune response in ways specific to the needs of the individual. *(3, 4)*

Anti-viral effects

Lactoferrin directly inhibits viruses by binding to viral receptor sites preventing the virus from infecting healthy cells. In vitro studies have demonstrated that lactoferrin strongly binds to receptors on HIV-1 and HIV-2, resulting in inhibition of virus-cell fusion and entry of the virus into cells. *(10)*

Lactoferrin also indirectly kills or inhibits viruses by augmenting the systemic immune response to a viral invasion. There is a systemic deficiency of lactoferrin in people with HIV infection. *(6, 11)* Lactoferrin was found to have "potent" anti-viral effects against the replication of both human HIV and cytomegalovirus (CMV) in several in vitro studies.

Studies have found that lactoferrin inhibits herpes simplex type 1 and type 2 infections of healthy cells. *(7 - 10, 16)*

Anti-microbial effects

Lactoferrin is a powerful anti-microbial that inhibits a wide range of pathogenic bacteria and other microbes. The mechanism appears to lie with lactoferrins' strong iron ability. Many pathogenic bacteria need a supply of free iron to multiply.

One study demonstrated that lactoferrin strongly inhibited helicobacter pylori in vitro and in vivo. *(12)* Another study demonstrated the effectiveness of lactoferrin as a natural anti-bacterial protein for preventing bacterial infections in mice. *(13)* Several studies have found lactoferrin to inhibit a wide range of gram positive and gram negative bacteria, yeasts, and even certain intestinal parasites including cholera, escherichia coli, shigella flexneri, staphylococcus epidermidis, pseudomonas aeruginosa, candida albicans, and others. *(14, 15)* There is also evidence that lactoferrin may improve the efficiency of anti-biotics.

Lactoferrin as an antioxidant

Lactoferrin is an antioxidant that scavenges free iron, helping to prevent iron based free radical reactions. Lactoferrin acts as both an iron binding agent and iron donor, depending on the physiological needs of the body. *(17)*

Anti-cancer effects

Extensive research with animals has shown lactoferrin to be a powerful anti-cancer agent both in vitro (test tube) and in vivo. Lactoferrin has been demonstrated to reduce the development of tumors from toxic chemical exposure and to reduce angiogenesis (the production of new blood vessels), which tumors need to grow. Metastasis to the lungs and liver was also suppressed and no adverse effects were observed. *(18 - 20)*

Lactoferrin also increased natural killer (NK) cell toxicity to several cancer cell lines at low concentrations. Lactoferrin was also found to suppress the growth of human pancreatic cancer cells. *(21, 18)*

Contraindications, Interactions & Precautions

Bovine lactoferrin has been determined to be "Generally Recognized as Safe" by the United States Food and Drug Administration for use as an ingredient in sports drinks and functional foods and is currently marketed in dietary supplement form. Because the highest concentration of human lactoferrin is found in breast milk (and tears), infants consume significant quantities of human lactoferrin, which has been proven to be safe. Humans have consumed bovine lactoferrin for thousands of years through cow's milk, where it is naturally found, which has been proven to be safe.

Some individuals may have a hypersensitivity or allergy to lactoferrin. It is contraindicated for those individuals.

38

Dosage and Administration of Lactoferrin

Oral lactoferrin, dosed at 40 mg daily, has been used in a couple of clinical trials of the substance. Those who supplement with lactoferrin typically take 250 mg daily.

Chapter 10 - Beta 1,3 Glucan

Beta glucan is a polysaccharide derived from the cell wall of baker's yeast, oat and barley fiber, and many medicinal mushrooms, such as Reishi, Shiitake, and Maitake. Yeast and mushrooms contain a mixture of beta 1,3 glucan and beta 1,6 glucan. Oats and barley contain a mixture of beta 1,3 glucan and beta 1,4 glucan. Some products may be listed as beta 1,3 1,6 glucan in the case of yeast-derived products and as beta 1,3 1,4 glucan when derived from oats.

Beta Glucan Enhances Immune Function

Literally hundreds of studies have shown that beta 1,3 glucan in particular activates macrophages and neutrophils. Exactly which molecular versions of beta 1,3 glucans are more effective and which sources are best is unclear.

Macrophages are the oldest and most primitive of the immune system components and provide one of the first lines of defense against infectious organisms. Macrophages recognize, engulf, and digest invading microorganisms, cellular debris, and cancer cells. They are the "pac men" of the immune system. (1 - 6) In addition to the activation of macrophages, it appears that beta 1,3 glucan also has receptors on human dermal fibroblasts. It appears that some of the beta 1,3 functional activity may be due to its interaction with non-immune cells in the body. (10)

Beta 1,3 glucans appear to have immune modulation effects on a broad scale. Some studies show that beta 1, 3 glucans increase the production of cytokines such as tumor necrosis factor and certain subsets of T-lymphocytes. These results suggest that beta 1,3 glucans enhance both non-specific host defense and cellular immune response. (7, 8) Toxins from infections cause leukocytes to release pro-inflammatory cytokines that can produce a series of biochemical events that ends in septic shock. Administration of soluble beta-1,3 glucans reduces the production of pro-inflammatory cytokines, which reduces mortality. (9)

Beta 1,3 Glucan Protects Against Radiation Exposure

In a controlled study done at the US Armed Forces Radiobiology Institute, 70% of rats given a lethal dose of radiation were completely protected from radiation effects when given a dose of yeast beta glucan by mouth after the radiation exposure. Beta glucan is a free radical scavenger. It is able to protect blood macrophages from free radical attack during and after the radiation allowing these cells to continue to function in the irradiated body and release factors important to the restoration of normal bone marrow production. *(11, 12)*

Beta Glucan Lowers Cholesterol

Beta glucan is the key factor for the cholesterol lowering effect of oat bran. *(13 - 17)* As with other soluble-fiber components, the binding of cholesterol by beta glucan and the resulting elimination of these molecules in the feces helps reduce blood cholesterol levels. *(18 - 20)* Results from a number of double-blind trials with either oat or yeast derived beta glucan indicate typical reductions, after at least four weeks of use, of approximately 10% for total cholesterol and 8% for LDL ("bad") cholesterol, and elevations in HDL ("good") cholesterol ranging from zero to 16%. *(21 - 25)*

Beta Glucans Reduce Glycemic Effect

Like other sources of soluble fiber, beta glucan is helpful in reducing the elevation in blood sugar levels that typically follow a meal. *(26 - 29)* Beta glucan reduces the elevation of blood sugar by delaying gastric emptying so that dietary sugar is absorbed more gradually.

Beta Glucan Dosage

Beta 1,3 glucans do not occur naturally in humans. There is no established minimum daily requirement.

For lowering cholesterol levels, the amount of beta glucan used in clinical trials has ranged from 2,900 to 15,000 mg per day. For enhancing immune function, an effective amount has not yet been determined. Manufacturers of beta glucan products usually recommend between 50 and 1,000 mg daily.

For best results, beta 1,3 glucans should be taken on an empty stomach. Beta 1,3 glucans are transported across the intestinal cell wall into the lymph where they begin to interact with macrophages to activate immune function. *(30)* Studies have verified that both small and large fragments of beta glucans are found in the serum, indicating that they are absorbed from the intestinal tract. *(31)*

Beta Glucan Safety and Side Effects

Although side effects are rare, occasionally an allergic reaction is reported. *(32, 33)*

Beta glucans are Generally Recognized as Safe (GRAS) by the FDA. Beta glucans are considered safe and non-toxic. *(34)*

Chapter 11 - Thymic Protein A

The thymus gland is the core of the human immune system. The thymus gland shrinks as we age. This shrinkage corresponds to a decline in immune function. *(5)*

In our early twenties we have an abundance of well functioning T-cells that regulate the immune system and help the body fight off pathogens and disease. Over time, our thymus gland shrinks and the output of thymic hormones decreases significantly. It is the gradual loss of thymic hormone and functioning T-cells that is thought to be responsible for many of the age-related changes in the immune system.

Animal extracts and synthetic thymic hormones have demonstrated the ability to dramatically reverse thymic atrophy and restore levels of immunity to much more youthful levels. Thymic extracts and thymic hormones are also among the few agents that are documented to extend the life span of experimental animals. *(7, 8)*

Thymic Protein A was first discovered and isolated by Terry Beardsley, Ph.D., an immunologist and experimental biologist from Baylor College of Medicine in Texas. Dr. Beardsley is considered one of the leading experts in the world on the thymus gland. After much research Dr. Beardsley discovered a complete, biologically "intact" 500-amino chain protein that fits into the receptor sites on T-4 cells to "turn on" and program the cells for their disease fighting functions. He named this peptide Thymic Protein A. Dr. Beardsley further developed an oral delivery system to avoid the protein degradation that occurs in the stomach. *(9 - 12)*

Since Thymic Protein A was introduced as an oral nutritional supplement, thousands of individuals have consumed this product. Hundreds of medical doctors are using it for a variety of immune-related illnesses with no adverse reactions.

Thymic Protein A is protein that has been formulated for effective absorption through the sublingual mucosa. Thymic protein A is administered by placing a packet of powder under the tongue and holding it there where it is absorbed directly into the blood stream. Dosage recommendations vary, ranging from one to two packets per week to several packets per day. The effectiveness of the immune response to infections and pathogenic agents is determined, in part, by the number of T-cells that are functioning properly. The reported benefits of Thymic Protein A include increased stamina, energy, well being, and ability to ward off infections. *(1, 5, 6)*

For best results, general supplementation with a complete vitamin mineral supplement is recommended. Vitamins A and C and Zinc in particular are known for their immune system support roles. It is reasonable to assume that the effectiveness of thymic protein A will be enhanced when these immune system supporting nutrients are present in optimum levels.

Chapter 12 - Cimetidine

Cimetidine is an over the counter drug that is a histamine 2 receptor antagonist that reduces stomach acid secretions and is marketed as a remedy for heart burn. It also suppresses the body's T cell suppressors. Normally the human immune system has some checks and balances built in to regulate its activity. If it is not aggressive enough, the body may suffer from infections or cancer. If it is too aggressive, the body may suffer from auto-immune disorders.

By temporarily suppressing the T cell suppressors, the immune system is up-regulated and rendered more active in attacking the infectious agents and cancer cells. Clinical studies published in peer reviewed medical and scientific journals have reported that cimetidine is as effective as anti-viral drugs in reducing the severity and duration of an outbreak of both herpes simplex and herpes zoster viruses. Cimetidine may be one of the most effective therapies for herpes simplex and herpes zoster outbreaks. (2 - 7, 15)

A ten day course of cimetidine costs approximately $10 while a ten day course of patented anti-viral drugs may run from $100 to $150.

Cimetidine has not been approved for the treatment of herpes virus infections. The approval and testing process is very costly and if approval was given, the result could be the replacement of expensive patented medicines with an inexpensive over the counter generic medicine.

In 1977, a patient being treated with cimetidine for a stomach ulcer experienced dramatic relief from a shingles outbreak that occurred at the same time. Subsequent tests with patients experiencing outbreaks of shingles, herpes labialis, and herpes keratitis demonstrated the effectiveness of cimetidine in reducing the severity and duration of the outbreaks. (2)

In 1996, a clinical study involving 221 patients with shingles demonstrated that cimetidine was effective in reducing the duration and severity of the outbreaks. The authors suggested using cimetidine in the early stages of the outbreak.*(3, 15)* A case reported in Canada resulted in the statement that cimetidine therapy appeared to reduce the expected length of the active phase of herpes zoster from 35 days or more to just 10 days. (4, 15)

Additional studies in Israel and Michigan State University confirmed that cimetidine shortened the median interval until the first decrease in pain, shortened the median interval until the complete resolution of pain, and promoted faster complete healing of skin lesions. *(5 - 7)*

The dosage that was used in the successful clinical trials was 200 mg three times daily and 400 mg at night. It has been suggested that cimetidine should be initiated as soon as the first symptoms of a herpes outbreak manifests and should be continued until the lesion disappears. It would not be prudent for one to take cimetidine continuously for prevention. *(3)*

In addition to the beneficial results for herpes simplex and herpes zoster, other studies have shown beneficial effects in the treatment of condylomata acuminata in children and indicated that cimetidine had a beneficial effect on genital warts. *(10)*

There have been numerous studies that suggest that cimetidine is useful as an anti-cancer agent. Apparently, cimetidine not only improves therapy outcomes by non-specifically boosting the immune system, but also facilitates the entry of killer lymphocytes into tumors and inhibits histamine which acts as a tumor growth and metastasis factor.

The literature reports positive results with several types of cancer but not all types. If interested, research the literature for the specific type of cancer of interest. A number of citations are included in the references.

Possible food and drug interactions with Cimetidine

If Cimetidine is taken with certain other drugs, the effects of either can be increased, decreased, or altered. It is especially important that you check with your doctor before combining cimetidine with any medication. A partial list of drugs that interact with cimetidine include the following:

- Anti-diabetic drugs such as Micronase and Glucotrol
- Antifungal drugs such as Diflucan and Nizoral
- Aspirin
- Augmentin
- Benzodiazepine tranquilizers such as Valium and Librium
- Beta-blocking blood pressure drugs such as Inderal and Lopressor
- Calcium-blocking blood pressure drugs such as Cardizem, Calan, and Procardia
- Chlorpromazine (Thorazine)
- Cisapride (Propulsid)
- Cyclosporine (Sandimmune)
- Digoxin (Lanoxin)
- Medications for irregular heartbeat, such as Cordarone, Tonocard, Quinidex, and Procan
- Metoclopramide (Reglan)
- Metronidazole (Flagyl)
- Narcotic pain relievers such as Demerol and Morphine
- Nicotine (Nicoderm, Nicorette)
- Paroxetine (Paxil)
- Pentoxifylline (Trental)
- Phenytoin (Dilantin)
- Quinine
- Sucralfate (Carafate)
- Theophylline (Theo-Dur, others)
- Warfarin (Coumadin)

Avoid alcoholic beverages while taking cimetidine. Cimetidine increases the effects of alcohol. Other antacids can reduce the effect of cimetidine when taken at the same time. If you take an antacid to relieve the pain of an ulcer, the doses should be separated by 1 to 2 hours. *(55)*

Before taking Cimetidine

Tell your doctor and pharmacist if you are allergic to cimetidine or any other medications. Tell your doctor and pharmacist what prescription and nonprescription medications, vitamins, nutritional supplements, and herbal products you are taking. Your doctor may need to change the doses of your medications or monitor you carefully for side effects.

If you are taking antacids (Maalox, Mylanta, Tums), digoxin (Lanoxin), ketoconazole (Nizoral), or iron salts, take them 2 hours before cimetidine.

Tell your doctor if you have or have ever had human immunodeficiency virus (HIV), acquired immunodeficiency syndrome (AIDS), or kidney or liver disease.

Tell your doctor if you are pregnant, plan to become pregnant, or are breast-feeding. If you become pregnant while taking cimetidine, call your doctor. *(55)*

Cimetidine Side Effects

Cimetidine may cause side effects. If you take Cimetidine tell your doctor if any of these symptoms are severe or do not go away:

- headache
- diarrhea
- dizziness
- drowsiness
- breast enlargement

Some side effects can be serious. The following symptoms are uncommon, but if you experience any of them, call your doctor immediately:

- confusion
- excitement
- depression
- nervousness

- seeing things or hearing voices that do not exist (hallucinating)

Cimetidine may cause other side effects. Call your doctor if you have any unusual problems while taking this medication. *(55)*

Cimetidine Dosage

The dosage that was used in the successful clinical trials was 200 mg three times daily plus 400 mg at night. Anyone who chooses to take Cimetidine with or against medical advice should consult a physician regarding their actions to obtain a diagnosis, advice on alternative treatments, and advice on possible drug interactions.

Chapter 13 - Coconut Oil and Monolaurin

Coconut Oil and Monolaurin have anti-viral properties. Coconuts and coconut oil have been traditional, staple foods of Asia, Africa, Central America, and the Pacific Islands for thousands of years. Pacific islanders, those who still eat traditional diets, have a reputation for good health and strong beautiful bodies. Many of these traditional diets obtain 30% to 60% of their calories from coconuts and coconut oil. They tend to have normal cholesterol levels and no cardiovascular disease. *(39)*

Prior to the early 1900's, coconut oil was the principal dietary fat in the United States. At that time cardiovascular disease was relatively uncommon. Subsequently, coconut oil has virtually disappeared, replaced by soybean oil, corn oil, and canola oil and the hydrogenated versions of these oils. While these domestic oils and their synthetic derivatives are under suspicion of causing a host of health problems, coconut oil research is revealing multiple health benefits for this oil.

Today, in countries where coconut oil is still widely used, heart and vascular disease remains uncommon.

Coconut oil is converted, by the body, into the hormone pregnenolone. It also has immune-stimulating and anti-oxidant action. Coconut oil also promotes thermogenesis and increased metabolism (possibly by supporting thyroid and mitochondrial function).

Coconut Oil and Cholesterol

Although coconut oil is a saturated fat, research has shown that it has a neutral effect on cholesterol and triglyceride levels. Being a saturated fat, it is stable and not oxidized easily, probably explaining why it does not contribute to coronary heart disease. *(3, 5, 12, 15, 31, 32, 34 - 38, 44, 48, 49)*

Coconut Oil - Immune Support and Antibiotic Properties

Two thirds of coconut oil consists of Medium Chain Triglycerides. These MCTs consist of lauric acid (48 percent), capric acid (7 percent), and caprylic acid (8 percent). These fatty acids and their monoglycerides are extremely powerful

50

antimicrobial agents, effective against a broad range of pathologic bacteria, viruses, fungi, yeasts, and protozoa.

The antiviral properties of lauric acid was first discovered when researchers were investigating the anti-infective properties of human breast milk. Human and mammalian breast milk is rich in lauric acid. These fatty acids and monoglycerides provide protection against infections to babies, whose immune systems are still developing. *When nursing mothers include coconut oil in their diet, the level of these fatty acids in their breast milk can triple.* (6, 18, 20 - 22, 28, 45, 52)

Anti-Viral Mechanism of Coconut Oil and Monolaurin

The monoglycerides have antiviral properties, diglycerides and triglycerides do not. Of the saturated fatty acids, lauric acid has greater antiviral activity than either caprylic acid or myristic acid. It has been reported that monolaurin is more effective in inactivating viruses and other infective agents than lauric acid. The exact difference between coconut oil and monolaurin as an anti-infective agent is unclear because they have not been adequately tested and studied. Most of the clinical studies have been done on Monolaurin. Monolaurin is a glyceride ester derivative of lauric acid; an activated form of lauric acid.

Monolaurin dissolves the lipids and phospholipids in the envelope of the virus causing the disintegration of the virus envelope effectively lysing the plasma membrane. There is also evidence that signal transduction is also interfered with, inhibiting the multiplication of the virus. (9, 16, 18, 21, 22, 51)

Viruses Inactivated by Coconut Oil

Some of the viruses inactivated by these lipids are HIV, measles virus, herpes simplex virus-1 (HSV-1), herpes simplex virus-2 (HSV-2), vesicular stomatitis virus (VSV), visna virus, and cytomegalovirus (CMV). Many of the pathogenic organisms reported to be inactivated by these antimicrobial lipids are those known to be responsible for opportunistic infections in HIV-positive individuals. In addition to viruses, several bacteria and fungi have also been reported to be suppressed by monolaurin and coconut oil. (1, 11, 14, 22, 24, 26, 27, 33, 40, 43, 45, 46, 50, 51)

Coconut Oil - Thermogenesis and Weight Loss

Research has shown that coconut oil increases thermogenesis, the rate of burning calories to produce heat and energy from food. Research has also shown that animals fed MCT oils had smaller fat pads and a number of key adipogenic genes were down-regulated. MCT fed animals also had improved insulin sensitivity, glucose tolerance and reduced adipose tissue lipoprotein lipase.

It has become clear that individuals consuming coconut oil rather than soybean or other LCT (long chain triglyceride) oils have an edge in losing weight and keeping it off. (2, 10, 15, 30, 44, 48, 49)

Organic Virgin Coconut Oil

There are basically two grades of coconut oil available: RBD (refined, bleached, and deodorized) and virgin coconut oil. RBD oil is subjected to high heat, filtration, and processed with sodium hydroxide. A properly produced RBD oil is an acceptable food product.

The ultimate coconut oil is organic, virgin coconut oil. The lauric acid content typically runs 50-55 percent making it a particularly potent antimicrobial. This oil has a distinct coconut smell and taste where RBD oil is usually bland, with no coconut taste or odor.

How to Use Coconut Oil

You can use coconut oil for all frying and stir frying. It is heat stable and has a shelf life of over one year at room temperature. You can also use it as a direct substitute for butter, ghee, margarine and other culinary oils. When warmed (it needs to be liquefied, it solidifies at 70 degrees F) and combined with a culinary vinegar and herbs, it makes an excellent salad dressing.

Dosage: How much (Coconut Oil) lauric acid or Monolaurin is needed?

Infants probably consume between 0.3 and 1 gram per kilogram of body weight if they are fed human milk or an enriched infant formula that contains coconut oil. This amount appears to have always been protective to some degree. Extrapolating breast milk content of lauric acid and scaling the quantity to the body weight of an adult, an estimated intake of approximately **24 grams of coconut oil** per day may provide protective levels for an adult. This is the equivalent of **3.5 tablespoons of coconut oil, 10 ounces of coconut milk** or **7 ounces of raw coconut** (approximately **one half of a raw coconut** per day).

The Dayrit (8) study of Monolaurin and coconut oil as a therapy for HIV used dosages of 7.5 to 22 grams of monolaurin per day in three divided doses or 45 ml. (approximately 3 tablespoons) of coconut oil per day. The coconut oil and monolaurin both demonstrated a beneficial result in reducing viral loads and improving white cell counts. Growing children probably need about the same amount as adults.

Safety Precautions and Side Effects

Coconut oil is food and can be consumed freely without any adverse effects. The only precaution is to keep your total calories within the range that is appropriate for your body type and activity level. Lauric acid from coconut oil is converted into monolaurin in the human body. Monolaurin is also considered to be a food.

Chapter 14 - BHT

BHT has anti-viral properties and may also limit inflammation through its action as an anti-oxidant. BHT is a synthetic antioxidant and common food preservative, approved by the FDA for food, oils, and fats. Over 25 years ago, a paper was published in the journal <u>Science</u> showing that BHT could inactivate herpes simplex and other lipid coated viruses in vitro (In lab dishes). *(1)* This was followed by another paper published in <u>Science</u> showing that BHT could prevent chickens from dying of Newcastle disease. *(2)* The herpes virus and the virus that causes Newcastle's disease both have a lipid envelope. That is, the nucleic acid core of these viruses is coated with a fatty membrane. Viruses of this type require an intact lipid membrane in order to penetrate cell walls and infect living cells.

BHT appears to work against such viruses by disrupting their lipid membranes making them vulnerable to the immune system and imparting their ability to penetrate human cells. BHT also removes binding proteins that the virus uses to penetrate cell membranes. In addition, BHT acts as an antioxidant neutralizing free radicals that damage cell membranes and cause inflammation. It is believed that the destructive action of many pathogenic viruses involves the destructive action of free radicals on cellular membranes.

More recent studies have confirmed the anti-viral activity of BHT against many different human and animal viruses including CMV (cytomegalovirus), *(3)* pseudo rabies *(4)*, genital herpes *(5)*, HIV *(6)*, and some strains of influenza. *(7)* A few of the viruses that have a lipid envelope, and may be affected by BHT, include herpes simplex I, herpes simplex II, herpes zoster, cytomegalovirus, west Nile virus, HIV virus, influenza virus, hepatitis B and C viruses, avian flu influenza virus, and the SARS virus. Remember that BHT has not been clinically tested and approved to treat these infections.

Based on these early scientific results, some individuals afflicted with herpes virus infections began experimenting on themselves with BHT. They used dosages in the 250 to 3000 mg per day range with the result that they experienced a reduction in herpes outbreaks. For some, their eruptions remained suppressed for as long as they continued to take BHT daily. For others, they were able to eventually discontinue taking BHT with no recurrences. BHT is discussed in Mann and Fowke's book, "Wipe Out Herpes with BHT," and Pearson and Shaw's book, "Life Extension." *(8, 9)*

At issue is that none of the controlled studies on the antiviral properties of BHT have been performed on humans. Rather, most of the experiments have been conducted in the laboratory or on animals. In addition, BHT is a common, inexpensive substance that is unpatentable. No pharmaceutical company will invest money in researching and certifying its value as a medication. Furthermore, it may be difficult to perform human trials because the Food and Drug Administration (FDA) has approved BHT for use only as a food preservative, not as a medicine.

Therefore, it is not approved for the treatment of herpes infections or any other disease. While doctors have the authority to prescribe BHT, they could face peer pressure and malpractice insurance issues for using an unapproved treatment. Your doctor may be reluctant to recommend or prescribe BHT. If you decide to make an independent decision to take BHT, at least tell your doctor what you are doing so that he can give you advice regarding your diagnosis, your other treatment options, potential consequences, possible drug interactions, etc.

The lack of approval hasn't stopped some people from using BHT on their own to treat herpes or other viral conditions. While there is no accounting of how many people have used BHT to treat herpes and other viral infections, the estimates run from thousands to hundreds of thousands.

BHT Safety Concerns and Side Effects

Studies performed on rats demonstrated liver and kidney damage at doses of 0.5 to 1.0 grams per kilogram of body weight. *(10)* This is the equivalent of a 160 pound adult taking 73 grams per day. Compare this to a typical suppressing dose of 0.25 to 0.50 grams per day and a typical dosage for an acute outbreak of 1.0 to 2.0 grams per day.

No evidence was noted for BHT causing cancer and conflicting results were obtained regarding effects on the immune system, tumor formation, and other effects. Again, all of these tests were done on rats and usually using high doses far in excess of therapeutic dosages.

BHT is metabolized by the liver and some of the rat experiments showed a suppression of liver enzymes and enlargement of the liver. This implies a degree of liver toxicity if the dose is high enough. At what dose a human might experience some degree of liver toxicity is unclear. Liver toxicity is a common side effect of a great many medications including some common over the counter pain relievers. If you are taking BHT or choose to take BHT, consider asking your doctor to do a blood test to measure your liver enzymes.

A large number of individuals have taken BHT in therapeutic doses for extended periods of time with no reported adverse effects. *(8, 9)* A case was reported in The New England Journal of Medicine of a patient who took 4 grams of BHT as a single dose on an empty stomach and experienced severe gastric pain, nausea, vomiting, and dehydration. *(11)* To be fair, a number of substances including aspirin, vitamin and mineral supplements, some foods, and many common medications can produce similar effects when taken on an empty stomach.

Additional anecdotal reports indicated that BHT may cause hives in a few individuals who are sensitive to BHT. BHT was also observed to temporarily cause a decrease in blood clotting when individuals first begin taking it in substantial doses. One individual reported dizziness and disorientation when taking 3 grams per day. His symptoms disappeared when he dropped his dose down to 250 mg per day. *(8, 9)*

There are a few physicians who regularly prescribe BHT for herpes treatment and outbreak prevention and consider it safe. There have been no formal clinical trials on humans to definitively determine the safety status of BHT.

BHT Dosage

Based on anecdotal information, it appears that a dosage of 250 mg to 1000 mg per day may be effective for many people. Dr. Ward Dean, M.D. recommends a dosage of 250 to 500 mg per day as an anti-oxidant and 2000 mg per day in divided doses for acute herpes outbreaks. *(12)*

BHT Precautions

- No one knows if there are any yet unrecognized health risks of large doses of BHT.

- Patients with diseases that compromise liver function should have their liver enzymes monitored by a physician.

- BHT is fat-soluble, so thin people may need less and may be more susceptible to side effects.

- BHT can interfere with blood clotting. It may pose a risk to persons with clotting problems or persons using anti-coagulant medications.

- Doses of BHT should start small and gradually increase.

- A few people are chemically sensitive to BHT.

- Alcohol should be avoided for at least several hours before and after taking BHT. Alcohol may have a stronger effect than usual.

- BHT can interact with some drugs. Check with your doctor or pharmacist regarding possible drug interactions before taking BHT.

- BHT is best taken with food, both to minimize any possible GI distress and to facilitate absorption.

- Anyone who chooses to take BHT with or against medical advice should consult a physician to obtain a diagnosis, advice on alternative treatments, and advice on possible drug interactions.

Chapter 15 - Lysine for Herpes

Lysine supplements and diets high in lysine and low in arginine have been used to discourage herpes outbreaks. Tissue culture studies have demonstrated that lysine inhibits viral replication. Analysis of the herpes simplex virons shows them to be rich in arginine and relatively lower in other essential amino acids including lysine. It appears that increasing the availability of lysine inhibits the utilization of arginine and slows virus replication. Experiments using Lysine supplements have shown that the intensity and frequency of outbreaks is reduced and quicker resolution of lesions is achieved.

The effectiveness of Lysine supplementation in suppressing herpes virus outbreaks is highly dose dependent, with beneficial effects apparent only at doses exceeding 1000 mg per day. One study indicated a decrease in recurrence rates in patients at a dose of 1248 mg of lysine monohydrochloride, but no effect at 624 mg daily. This study did not show any evidence of shortening the healing time compared to placebo. *(10)* Another small randomized controlled trial indicated the benefit of 3000 mg lysine daily for the reduction of occurrence, severity, and healing time for recurrent HSV infection. *(11, 12)*

In one study, serum lysine levels were measured. *(1)* It was determined that when a person's serum lysine concentration exceeded 165 nmol/ml there was a corresponding significant decrease in recurrence rate. Conversely, the frequency rate increased significantly as concentration levels fell below 165 nmol/ml. These results suggest that prophylactic lysine may be useful in managing selected cases of recurrent herpes simplex labialis if serum lysine levels can be maintained at adequate concentrations. Those studies that did not report positive results may not have used a high enough dose of lysine to be effective or the participants may have had a diet high in arginine.

It is also likely that arginine levels have an effect on results as well. If one wishes to suppress herpes virus growth with lysine supplements, it may be necessary to restrict arginine in the diet as well to keep the lysine to arginine ration in a favorable range. A list of foods with the arginine, lysine content and the arginine lysine ratio is contained in Appendix A.

It should also be noted that the studies that recorded positive results noted a reduction in the frequency of outbreaks and duration of outbreaks, not a complete suppression of outbreaks. This suggests that while lysine appears to be a useful therapy, best results may be obtained by combining it with additional therapies, either natural or orthodox.

Given that arginine is an essential amino acid and has important roles in endocrine function, long term arginine restriction may not be the best practice. Other treatment options may be more effective and desirable.

Chapter 16 - Garlic

Plants do not have immune systems to defend themselves against the bacteria, fungi, viruses, and yeasts that attack them. Their defense is direct chemical warfare. Their weapons are antibiotics, antivirals, and fungicides that they manufacture internally. Their success is demonstrated by the fact that you see healthy growing plants everywhere.

In the case of garlic, one of the main active ingredients is a thiosulfinate compound called allicin. The manufacture of allicin is triggered by the release of enzymes by breaking the cell walls of the garlic plant. Allicin is the pungent, hot, stinky stuff that makes garlic special. *(30)*

In addition to allicin, garlic contains over 100 other beneficial nutrients. These include beta-carotene, folate, beta-sitosterol, ferulic acid, geraniol, oleanolic acid, P-coumaric acid, rutin, quercetin, thiamine, niacin, vitamin c, cysteine, zinc, calcium, magnesium, manganese, selenium, and others. Some of the garlic compounds currently under investigation are: allin (responsible for the typical garlic odor), alline (odorless compound), ajoene (naturally occurring disulfide), diallyl sulfide (DAS), diallyl disulfide (DADS), diallyl trisulfide (DAT), S-allylcysteine (SAC), organosulfur compounds, and allyl sulfur compounds.

Garlic as an Anti-biotic and Anti-viral

In vitro (in laboratory cultures) studies demonstrate that garlic has antibacterial, antiviral, and antifungal activity. In one clinical study, one capsule daily of an allicin-containing garlic supplement was tested on a group of 146 volunteers (Josling P 2001). Over several months half the group received the garlic while the other half got a placebo. The placebo group had 63 percent more common cold infections than the garlic group. In addition, those in the garlic group who did catch a cold had symptoms for an average of only 1.52 days, compared with 5.01 days for the placebo group. The doctors who conducted this garlic study concluded, "An allicin-containing supplement can prevent attack by the common cold virus." *(28)* In addition, test tube studies have shown that garlic has antibacterial, antiviral, and antifungal activity. *(41)*

While these results are encouraging, garlic has not been clinically tested against many common infections.

Garlic in Herpes Virus Infections

While garlic has demonstrated in vitro anti-viral activity against many viruses including HSV-1 and HSV-2, clinical trials on humans have not been performed. Garlic's in vitro success against these viruses and its demonstrated in vivo effectiveness against the common cold virus suggest that it may be effective against the herpes viruses in humans as well. However, this hypothesis has not been clinically tested. *(26, 27, 28, 29, 41)*

Garlic for Lowering Blood Pressure

There is some evidence that garlic is mildly hypotensive in humans. Researchers at the University of Mississippi and in Turkey performed clinical tests on the effectiveness of garlic in reducing blood pressure. They found that garlic reduced systolic blood pressure by at least 9 mmHg and diastolic blood pressure by at least 5 mmHg. The effect was most noted in subjects with high blood pressure and high cholesterol. No hypotensive effect was observed in patients with normal blood pressure. *(11, 32, 60, 38)*

Garlic for Lowering Cholesterol

There is contradictory evidence as to whether garlic actually lowers cholesterol and triglyceride levels or not. The contradictions appear to arise from the use of different dosages, forms of garlic, and other procedural differences. However, most findings showed that garlic slightly lowered blood cholesterol, LDL cholesterol, and triglycerides with a consistent lowering of blood lipids seen in studies that used aged garlic extract (kyolic) as the supplement. Research has demonstrated that garlic inhibits the peroxidation of lipids. This, in turn, prevents LDL cholesterol from being oxidized into harmful compounds. Garlic also lowers homocysteine levels. Recent research has identified homocysteine as a

62

major culprit in heart disease, osteoporosis, alzheimers and several other degenerative diseases. *(25, 30 - 37)*

Garlic in Atherosclerosis

Garlic reduces platelet aggregation, thrombin formation, platelet adhesion to fibrinogen and the risk of thrombosis.   Garlic's effects are attributed to allicin, ajoene, and other organosulfur constituents in the herb. A recent study on garlic confirms that it exhibits powerful fibrinolytic activity both in vitro and in vivo. In this study, it acted as an anticoagulant by down regulating thrombin formation. These effects reduce the formation of atherosclerotic plaque.

In one study, patients with atherosclerosis, plasma levels of the oxidant MDA (malondialdehyde) were higher, and plasma levels of the antioxidant enzyme glutathione peroxidase were lower compared to the control group. However, those patients who consumed 1 ml/kg of garlic extract had significantly lowered MDA levels even in the absence of changes in antioxidant enzyme activities. In addition, the researchers found the presence of oxidant stress in blood samples from atherosclerosis patients, but ingesting garlic extract prevented oxidation reactions by eliminating this oxidant stress. *(9, 10, 24, 37, 51, 40)*

Garlic and Men's Health

Garlic may reduce the risk of prostate cancer, according to a recent study. Researchers surveyed 238 men with prostate cancer and 471 healthy controls in Shanghai, China to determine their eating habits. The risk of prostate cancer declined by more than 33 percent in men who consumed small amounts of onions, garlic, scallions, shallots and leeks each day. Men who consumed 2 grams of garlic daily experienced a 50 percent decease in prostate cancer risk. *(23)* Another study done with rats demonstrated that garlic supplementation in combination with a high protein diet increased testosterone levels.

Anti-Cancer Properties of Garlic

Modern epidemiological studies, well correlated with laboratory investigations, corroborate the evidence that higher intake of garlic and its relatives are correlated with reduced risk of several cancers. The mechanisms proposed to explain the cancer-preventive effects of garlic include inhibition of tumor mutagenesis, modulation of enzyme activities, and effects on cell proliferation and tumor growth.

Several garlic compounds, including allicin, induce apoptosis (programmed cell death) in various malignant human cells. These include breast, colorectal, hepatic, prostate, and lymphoma cells. A growing number of clinical studies are examining the properties of ajoene, one of the major components of purified garlic. Researchers are investigating Ajoene in part because it is more chemically stable than allicin.

The list of cancers responding to garlic treatment or supplementation continues to grow. The list currently includes basal cell carcinoma, chronic myeloid leukemia, some human bladder, liver and colon cancers. *(13 - 20, 39, 42, 43)*

How much is usually taken?

People who wish to consume garlic and have no aversion to its odor can chew from one to two whole cloves of raw garlic daily. In certain regions of China up to eight cloves of raw garlic are consumed per day. For those who prefer it with less odor, enteric-coated tablets or capsules with approximately 1.3% allin are available. Clinical trials have used 600–900 mg (delivering approximately 5–6 mg of allicin) per day in two or three divided amounts. Aged-garlic extracts have been studied in amounts ranging from 2.4–7.2 grams per day. *(44, 45)*

Garlic Side Effects and Drug Interactions

Garlic has anti-coagulant properties. Anyone with a bleeding disorder or taking anti-coagulant anti-platelet medications should consult their doctor before consuming garlic. Anyone anticipating surgery, child birth, etc., should avoid garlic because of the increased probability of bleeding.

Other side effects from garlic may include upset stomach, bloating, bad breath, and body odor. Garlic is considered to have very low toxicity and is listed as Generally Recognized as Safe (GRAS) by the Food and Drug Administration (FDA) of the United States. More research with better designed studies is needed in order to fully assess the safety and effectiveness of garlic and to determine the most appropriate dose and form. *(61 - 66)*

Garlic may reduce blood levels of protease inhibitors. Protease Inhibitors are a class of drugs used to treat people with the human immunodeficiency virus (HIV). They include indinavir, ritinavir, and saquinavir. *(67)* Anyone taking any of this class of medications should consult their physician before taking garlic supplements or eating garlic.

Author's Comments

If you dig deeply into the research on garlic, you will find a lot of published studies. Some of these studies yield results that are contradictory or inconsistent with others. It is this author's opinion that differences in outcomes are most likely the result of the use of non-standard garlic products. It is generally known that the concentration of active ingredients varies widely with different garlic supplements. It is also generally known that the body's ability to absorb the active ingredients contained in different supplements also varies. More conclusive studies would result if the researchers would correlate the actual blood levels of absorbed ingredients with the other experimental parameters.

It is possible that the best therapeutic effect may be obtained from eating fresh raw garlic rather than taking supplements.

Chapter 17 - Propolis

Propolis is produced by bees and is used as a construction material in bee hives. To protect the hive and its nutritious contents from attack by micro-organisms, propolis has anti-microbial properties. Propolis is comprised of a complex of chemicals (especially flavonoids), which play a role as antiviral and antibacterial agents. The composition of propolis can vary widely depending on the climate, season, species of bees, and other variables.

Propolis for Herpes

When propolis was administered to various laboratory animals and to Vero cells in vitro, significant inhibitory effects against HSV-1 were found. Propolis (5%) prevented development of symptoms of intraperitoneal HSV-1 infection in rats and corneal HSV-1 infection in rabbits. In one study, 90 men and women with recurrent genital HSV2 were divided into two groups to compare the healing ability of propolis ointment versus acyclovir ointment and placebo. At day 10, 80 percent of patients in the propolis group had healed versus 47 percent in the acyclovir group and 40 percent in the placebo group. *(4, 5, 9, 10, 25, 27)*

Human trials as an internal anti-viral agent have not been done. Based on successful laboratory and animal studies, and successful use as a topical agent on herpes lesions, it is hypothesized that it may be beneficial as an oral anti-viral agent in humans as well.

Anti-Bacterial & Anti-Viral Properties of Propolis

The early research on propolis was mostly done in Eastern Europe and the former Soviet Union. Laboratory tests demonstrated that propolis, on its own, is effective against over 20 kinds of bacteria. Clinical studies also demonstrated that propolis was effective against various kinds of bacterial, fungal, and viral infections. Dr. Kravcuk of Kiev found that propolis was effective against sore throats and dry coughs in 90% of 260 patients. A recent study by Serkedjieva, et al, showed that the active ingredients in propolis significantly inhibited the Hong Kong flu virus. *(8)*

In a recent study, Egyptian researchers examined two types of propolis and found they exhibited antibacterial activity against the bacteria Staphylococcus aureus and Escherichia coli as well as the fungus candida albicans. In a March 2004 article in the Archives of Pediatric and Adolescent Medicine, an herbal formula containing echinacea, propolis, and vitamin C was tested on 430 children in a double blind placebo controlled study. The group treated with the herbal formula experienced a 55 percent reduction in the number of illness episodes compared with the placebo group. In treated children, the mean number of episodes per child was decreased by half and the mean number of days each child suffered from a fever was reduced by 62 percent. *(1)*

The antibacterial properties of propolis appear to be due to multiple mechanisms. Propolis inhibits bacterial growth by preventing cell division. It also disorganizes bacterial cytoplasm, cell membranes, and cell walls. Propolis causes partial bacteriolysis and inhibits protein synthesis. In addition, propolis appears to enhance the effectiveness of antibiotics such as penicillin and streptomycin.

Propolis and Immune Enhancement

In addition to providing direct anti-bacterial and anti-viral effects, propolis also stimulates the body's immune system. Propolis significantly activates macrophages, inhibits lipoxygenase activity, inhibits prostaglandin synthesis and produces anti-inflammatory effects. *(13 - 16, 23)*

Propolis in the Prevention and Treatment of Cancer

Propolis may also have value in the prevention and treatment of cancer. Caffeic acid phenethyl ester (CAPE), one of the active ingredients in propolis, has been shown to prevent cancer formation in animal models. It also showed strong cancer inhibitory effects against several colon cancers, melanoma, and glioblastoma. Propolis inhibits cancer cell growth by increasing the process of apoptosis (programmed cell death). *(17 - 21)*

Other Uses of Propolis

Studies indicate that it may be effective in treating skin burns. *(27 - 29)* Propolis is also a subject of recent dentistry research, since there is some evidence that propolis may actively protect against caries and other forms of oral disease, due to its antimicrobial properties. *(31 - 34)*

Propolis Safety

Propolis is a non toxic substance for most people and will not cause irritation when used as supplements or applied to skin.

However, like other honey bee products, there are people who are allergic to propolis. If you're allergic to propolis, it may cause your skin to redden, develop rashes, swell, itch, and may even lead your skin to crack. In addition, it may also irritate the skin area where it's applied on, cause eczema, lesions, psoriasis, or mouth sores.

Who could be potentially at risk of a propolis allergy? Here are a few possibilities.

- Those who have a known pollen allergy.

- Asthma patients may have an increased risk of allergic reactions in general.

- Those who are known to be allergic to bee stings.

- Pregnant women. There is no published information on the use of propolis in pregnancy.

- Those with known allergies to black poplar (also populas nigra), poplar buds, honey, and balsam of Peru. There are around 8 to 13 compounds that propolis and balsam of Peru have in common.

Individuals with allergies, especially allergies to bees, pollen, etc. should exercise caution and consult with their physician before using propolis.

The LD50 (a dose causing half of the tested animals to die) for propolis is 7.34 g/Kg of body weight in mice. That is close to 50 gm of propolis for a 160 pound person. Propolis has also been reported to be non-irritating and safe for topical use. *(24)*

Chapter 18 - Proteolytic Enzymes

Orally administered pancreatic enzyme preparations have been used for the treatment of inflammation, injuries, and shingles outbreaks for over 30 years. Inflammation is part of the body's normal healing response to injury and infections. However, severe injury or infection can trigger an inflammatory cascade that can cause complications, excessive pain, and hinder the healing process. Numerous studies have shown that proteolytic enzymes taken orally reduce pain and inflammation from injuries and surgery. *(10, 17 - 19)*

Proteolytic enzyme supplementation reduces inflammation by neutralizing bradykinins and pro-inflammatory eicosanoids to levels where the synthesis, repair, and regeneration of injured tissues can begin.

Absorption of Oral Proteolytic Enzymes

Enzymes are proteins and proteins are broken down by the digestive process into discrete amino acids. The question has been raised as to how orally administered enzymes could possibly get into the blood and produce a therapeutic effect. Early studies demonstrated therapeutic effects from proteolytic enzymes that were administered by injection. Later studies done in the 1950's and 1960's demonstrated that enterically coated proteolytic enzymes administered orally are absorbed into the blood and produce physiological effects. Studies were performed on papain, bromelain, chymotrypsin, and trypsin that were enterically coated. *(3 - 9)*

Enteric coating is a substance used to protect the enzymes from stomach acid but dissolve in the intestines and allow the enzymes to be absorbed intact through the intestinal wall.

Shingles - Herpes Zoster (Chicken Pox)

Proteolytic enzymes may be helpful for the initial attack of shingles. Shingles is caused by the herpes zoster virus, the same virus that causes chicken pox. A double-blind study of 190 people with shingles compared proteolytic enzymes to the antiviral drug acyclovir. Participants were

70

treated for 14 days and their pain was assessed at intervals. Both groups had similar pain relief, but the enzyme-treated group experienced fewer side effects. Another double-blind study in which 90 people were given either an injection of acyclovir or proteolytic enzymes followed by a course of oral medication for 7 days showed similar beneficial results. *(20, 21, 57 - 59)*

Additional studies have investigated the use of proteolytic enzymes as a treatment for other viral agents including HIV *(60)*, Hepatitis C *(61, 64)* and Hepatitis B *(62, 63)*. The results reported were generally positive but more research is needed.

Sports Injuries

A double-blind, placebo-controlled study of 44 people with sports-related ankle injuries found that treatment with proteolytic enzymes improved healing time by about 50%. *(22)* Three additional small double-blind studies, involving a total of about 80 athletes, found that treatment with proteolytic enzymes significantly improved the healing of bruises and other mild athletic injuries as compared to placebo. *(23 - 25)* Another study involving 71 individuals with finger fractures found that treatment with proteolytic enzymes improved recovery times. *(26)* In another double-blind trial, 100 people were treated for experimentally induced hematomas (bruises) with proteolytic enzymes. The researchers found that enzyme treatment significantly speeded recovery. *(27)*

Surgery

Numerous studies using several different proteolytic enzyme protocols with surgery patients have produced mixed results. The mixed results may represent the use of different enzyme protocols in the different studies. The use of mixed proteolytic enzymes was found to be beneficial in knee surgery, oral surgery, dental surgery, episotomy surgery, nasal surgery, foot surgery, and cataract removal. *(28 - 42)*

Chronic Musculoskeletal Pain

A double-blind, placebo-controlled trial of 30 people with chronic neck pain found that use of a proteolytic enzyme mixture modestly reduced pain symptoms as compared to a placebo. *(43)*

Proteolytic Enzymes and Osteoarthritis

A clinical trial demonstrated significant improvement for individuals with degenerative arthritis of the lower spine and sciatica-type leg pain. *(49, 50)* A study involving more than 300 people compared proteolytic enzymes to the standard anti-inflammatory medications for the treatment of osteoarthritis of the shoulder, back, or knee. The results showed equivalent benefits with the supplement and the medication. *(44, 45)*

Proteolytic enzymes in cancer therapy

The use of proteolytic enzymes for cancer treatment began with Scottish Embryologist John Beard. Beard noted the similarity between placenta cells and cancer cells and the regulation of the growth of both types of cells fetal pancreatic proteolytic enzymes. (Placenta cells are now called stem cells) He published his work in his book <u>The Enzyme Treatment of Cancer and its Scientific Basis</u>. Following Beard, proteolytic enzymes have been promoted by numerous alternative cancer practitioners. More recently Nicholas Gonzalez, M.D. is evaluating the benefit of proteolytic enzymes in patients with advanced pancreatic cancer in a large-scale study, funded by the National Institute of Health's National Center for Complementary and Alternative Medicine, with collaboration from the National Cancer Institute. This larger trial is a follow-up to a smaller study that showed dramatic positive results.

The clinical research that currently exists on proteolytic enzymes suggests significant benefits in the treatment of many forms of cancer. These studies have shown improvements in the general condition of patients with cancers of the breast, lung, stomach, head and neck, ovaries, cervix, and colon, along with lymphomas and multiple myeloma. These studies involved the use of proteolytic enzymes in conjunction with conventional therapy (surgery, chemotherapy and/or radiation). The results showed modest to significant improvements in quality of life and life expectancy. *(65, 66)*

Safety Issues

In some infrequent cases, proteolytic enzymes have been associated with digestive upset or allergic reactions. *(47)* In addition, pancreatin may interfere with folate absorption. *(46)* Papain and bromelain may have anti-coagulant properties and could complicate bleeding disorders or interfere with anti-coagulant medications. Bromelain may increase the blood concentration of certain anti-biotics and may interact with certain sedatives. *(47)* Individuals with malabsorption syndromes are often deficient in fat digesting lipases and, therefore, should use enzyme mixtures that are high in lipase and low in proteolytic enzymes because the proteolytic enzymes may destroy lipase. *(48)* Colon damage has been reported in children with cystic fibrosis who receive enzyme therapy. The exact mechanism and parameters are not clearly understood. Children with cystic fibrosis should avoid proteolytic enzymes until this issue is better understood. *(51 - 56)*

For the majority of individuals, oral proteolytic enzymes are considered quite safe.

Chapter 19 - Indole-3-Carbinol

Indole-3-carbinol or I3C is a breakdown product of glucosinolate glucobrassicin which is primarily found in cruciferous vegetables. Cruciferous vegetables include cabbage, broccoli, brussel sprouts, cauliflower, bok choy, and kale.

When cruciferous vegetables are macerated (cell walls broken), an enzyme called myrosinase is released. Myrosinase produces I3C from the glucosinolates in the vegetables. I3C is converted to diindolymethane (DIM), indole (3,2,b) carbazole (ICZ) and other compounds by stomach acid. DIM and ICZ are absorbed from the gastrointestinal tract. The most recent research attributes DIM as the primary anti-cancer compound.
Research indicates that Indole-3 carbinol and its derivatives may modulate estrogen metabolism and have anti-carcinogenic, antioxidant and anti-atherogenic properties. *(1)*

Indole-3 Carbinol and Herpes Viruses

Research has shown that I3C is a "cell cycle G1 antagonist" and that herpes simplex virus (HSV) requires cell cycle factors to replicate. Subsequently, an in vitro study investigated the effect of I3C on monkey kidney and human lung cells infected with HSV-1 and HSV-2 viruses. The replication of all HSV types tested was inhibited by at least 99.9% by the I3C but the test cells required pretreatment with I3C for at least 12 to 36 hours prior to infection. The observed inhibition was not due to direct viral inactivation by I3C or drug induced cytoxicity. Rather, inhibition was the apparent result of disrupting cell cycle factors required by HSV for replication. I3C may also be useful in inhibiting the formation of papillomatosis cysts caused by the human papilloma virus (HPV). *(2)*

There are some questions regarding the potential use of I3C as an anti-viral treatment. I3C is metabolized into its derivatives by stomach acid. It is unclear whether the derivatives or I3C itself is responsible for its anti-viral properties. If the derivatives should prove to be active anti-viral agents, then it may be possible to prevent herpes family viral outbreaks by daily consumption of I3C supplements, the derivatives, or substantial quantities of cruciferous vegetables.

Cancer, Indole-3 Carbinol and DIM

Historically, the Roman statesman, Cato the Elder (234 - 149 BC) wrote: "If a cancerous ulcer appears upon the breasts, apply a crushed cabbage leaf and it will make it well." Crushing a cabbage leaf would convert indole-3-glucosinolate to I3C, among other reactions. Recent research indicates that I3C and several of its derivatives, DIM in particular, modulate estrogen metabolism. Specifically, DIM increases the ratio of 2-hydroxyestrone to 16 alpha-hydroxyestrone and also inhibits the 4-hydroxylation of estradiol. *(3 - 6)*

This is important because 16 alpha-hydroxyestrone has been demonstrated to be carcinogenic while 2-hydroxylation has been demonstrated to have anti-cancer properties. Indole-3-carbinol has also been shown to increase apoptosis (cell death) in some cancer cell lines. I3C and DIM have demonstrated anti-cancer properties with endometrium, lung, tongue, colon, liver, breast, uterine and prostate cancers. DIM is also being investigated as a treatment for cervical dysplasia. *(7 - 9)*

Estrogen modulation is very important because many pesticides, plastics, and other synthetic chemicals in the environment mimic estrogen when introduced into the human body.

Increased estrogen levels from birth control pills can have undesirable health effects. Estrogen / testosterone imbalance associated with aging can contribute to age related weight gain and obesity. Imbalances in estrogen metabolites can increase the risk of certain cancers.

Some epidemiological studies involving humans have been done. In one study polish women were observed to have approximately four times the rate of breast cancer after immigrating to the United States. The increase in breast cancer was correlated with a reduction in the consumption of cruciferous vegetables, especially cabbage sauerkraut. It must be recognized that cruciferous vegetables are relatively good sources of other phytonutrients that may have protective effects against cancer, including vitamin C, folate, selenium, carotenoids, fiber, and a variety of glucosinolates that may be hydrolyzed to a variety of potentially protective isothiocyanates, in addition to indole-3-carbinol. It is possible that the anti-cancer effects of consuming cabbage sauerkraut may be the result of a combination of nutrients rather than I3C alone. *(10)*

Human Papilloma Virus

Human papilloma virus (HPV) infection is associated with an increased risk of cervical cancer, the second most common cancer in women and the seventh most common form of cancer worldwide. Fortunately, only a small percentage of women infected with HPV develop invasive cervical cancer. The evolution of HPV into cancer is triggered by estrogen.

Animal studies have demonstrated that I3C supplements reduce the risk of the development of cervical cancer in HPV infected animals. I3C has also been demonstrated to trigger cell death in precancerous cervical cells. *(11)*

Lupus

Researchers have discovered that women with Systemic Lupus Erythematosus (SLE) tend to metabolize estrogen through the disease-causing pathway, 16 alpha-hydroxylation. This opens the possibility that I3C may be beneficial to patients suffering from SLE. I3C and its derivative DIM have anti-estrogenic effects.

Twelve women with SLE took 375 mg/day of I3C for three months. The subjects' 16 alpha-hydroxylation activity decreased, the "tumor suppressor" 2-hydroxylation activity increased, and the disease activity index declined from 10.0 to 6.25. *(12)*

In a study using mice bred to develop lupus, I3C was fed to one group starting soon after birth. At 12 months of age, 80 percent of the I3C supplemented mice were alive compared to 10% of the control group. When the mice were given I3C beginning at five months of age, 100 percent of I3C fed mice and 30 percent of controls were alive one year later. *(13)*

I3C Drug Interactions

No drug interactions in humans have been reported. However, preliminary evidence suggests that that I3C and DIM can increase the activity of CYP1A2 and CYP3A4. CYP3A4 is involved in the metabolism of approximately 60% of therapeutic drugs. This suggests the possibility that I3C and DIM have the potential for adverse drug interactions. *(14 -16)*

The conversion of indole-3-carbinol to DIM and ICZ requires stomach acid. Therefore, antacids and stomach acid reducing medications may inhibit the effectiveness of I3C. Indole-3 carbinol may be synergistic with tamoxifen in protecting against breast cancer.

Indole-3 Carbinol from Food

The enzyme myrosinase is the key to obtaining maximum I3C and DIM from cruciferous vegetables. Enzymes are destroyed by cooking. Therefore, cruciferous vegetables provide the most I3C when consumed raw. The enzyme is released and activated by breaking the cell walls.

Therefore, bruising, macerating, crushing, blending, or otherwise mechanically disrupting as many cell walls as possible will yield the most I3C. There are two ways to meet this requirement. One is eating the vegetables raw and chewing them well. The other is making fermented vegetables. Traditional fermented sauerkraut uses exactly this process. Cabbage (or other cruciferous vegetables) is shredded and pounded, and then a small amount of salt is added to draw out the juice and provide an anaerobic environment for fermentation. The lactic acid produced by the fermentation facilitates conversion of I3C to DIM. Cruciferous vegetables are believed to have some goitrogenic properties which may be deactivated by fermentation as well.

The amount of raw cruciferous vegetables needed to provide a maximum protective benefit has been estimated to be a minimum of two pounds per day. Consuming this much is impractical. Research has indicated that individuals who consume a high amount of cruciferous vegetables in pre-teen and adolescent years retain a protective effect later in life, even if they no longer consume large amounts. Consumption later in life also provided a protective effect.

Indole-3 Carbinol Safety

Despite its overall anti-cancer effects, there is some evidence that I3C has tumor-promoting properties under certain circumstances. (17 - 19)

Indole-3-Carbinol activates many cellular enzymes and forms many derivative products. Some of these derivative products have been tested and produced mixed results with regards to benefits and safety. Given that epidemiological data shows that consumption of cruciferous vegetables is associated with health benefits, it would appear that I3C in reasonable nutritional quantities is not particularly hazardous. Taking high doses of I3C as a supplement may be another matter. The chemistry of I3C is quite complex. In brief, several derivative products are formed in the presence of stomach acid. Their acronyms are ICZ, LTR, CTR, ASG, and DIM. All of these except DIM have some beneficial and some harmful properties.

Only DIM exerts its control over cancer cell growth without activating the dioxin receptor or inducing unwanted enzymes. Direct control over cancer cell growth by DIM has now been shown in breast, uterine, cervical, ovarian, and colon cancer cells. It is believed that much of the anti-cancer activity attributed to I3C may be attributable to the DIM that forms from the I3C. DIM has, so far, a firmly established safety record and most current research with humans is focusing on DIM.

Slight increases in the liver enzyme ALT (alanine aminotransferase) were observed in two women who took unspecified doses of I3C for four weeks. (20)

One person reported a skin rash while taking 375 mg/day of I3C. (21)

78

High doses of I3C (800 mg/day) were associated with symptoms of disequilibrium and tremor, which resolved when the dose was decreased. *(22)*

I3C supplementation enhanced the development of cancer in some animal models when given after the carcinogen. *(23 - 26)*

DIM and Indole-3-Carbinol (I3C) Dosage

I3C is available without a prescription as a dietary supplement. I3C supplementation increased urinary 2OHE1 levels in adults at doses of 300-400 mg/day. *(27)*

I3C doses of 200 or 400 mg/day improved the regression of cervical intraepithelial neoplasia (CIN) in a preliminary clinical trial.

I3C in doses up to 400 mg/day has been used to treat recurrent respiratory papillomatosis. *(28, 29)*

DIM is available without a prescription as a dietary supplement.

In a small clinical trial, DIM supplementation at a dose of 108 mg/day for 30 days increased urinary 2OHE1 excretion in postmenopausal women with a history of breast cancer. *(30)*

Use of absorbable DIM has been shown effective in amounts close to that obtainable from our diet (0.3 mg/kg/day of DIM). That corresponds to 22 mg per day for a 160 pound individual. I3C requires about 15 times more than this (4.5 mg/kg/day), and may be associated with side effects. This corresponds to 327 mg per day for a 160 pound individual.

Chapter 20 - Resveratrol

Resveratrol is a naturally occurring substance that is found in the vines, roots, seeds, skins and stalks of grapes, peanuts, mulberries, the Japanese knotweed plant, and several other plants. Resveratrol, along with other polyphenols including quercetin, catechins, gallocatechins, procyanidins, and prodelphidins, are extracted from grape seeds and skins and found in red wine. Commercial resveratrol supplements generally obtain their resveratrol from the Japanese knotweed plant.

Resveratrol is a phytoalexin. It is produced by plants in response to injury or fungal infections as a defense against pathogens that would injure the plant. Resveratrol may have anti-microbial activity for humans as well. Research suggests that resveratrol may improve heart and cardiovascular health, reduce the risk of cancer, fight some infections, and increase the life span of humans.

Resveratrol and the Herpes Family Viruses

Resveratrol has shown activity against herpes simplex virus types 1 and 2 in a dose-dependent manner. It appears to disrupt a critical early event in the viral reproduction cycle. Resveratrol was found to inhibit herpes simplex virus types 1 and 2 replication by the direct inactivation of HSV, not inhibition of virus attachment to the cell. Resveratrol was most effective when added within 1 hour of cell infection, and not effective if added 9 hours post-infection. Resveratrol was also found to delay the cell cycle reproduction and inhibit reactivation of virus from latently infected neurons. These studies were performed on cells in vitro. (22, 23, 35)

Researchers also tested 19% resveratrol cream on skin and vaginal herpes lesions in mice and compared the results with topical acyclovir. The results were similar for both substances. (21)

Resveratrol and Life Extension

Recent research has demonstrated that resveratrol may trigger a genetic expression that facilitates extended life span. This is the same life extension effect that is associated with calorie restricted diets. Restricting calorie intake in laboratory animals has been shown to prolong their life span by as much as 60%. The same effect has not been proven in humans, but the research is ongoing and looks promising. Restricted calorie diets, however, lack popularity. The possibility that resveratrol may provide a similar benefit has caused considerable interest.

Recent studies show that resveratrol activates molecular pathways involved in life-span extension. This effect has now been demonstrated in yeast, worms, flies, fish, and mice. While this effect has not yet been demonstrated in humans, research is ongoing and looks promising. Research with mice also demonstrates that resveratrol mitigates the harmful effects of high calorie diets, including metabolic changes resembling diabetes, liver, and heart damage, and premature death. Resveratrol may enhance health and support longevity via multiple mechanisms, including potent antioxidant effects, enhancement of cellular energy production and influence of gene expression patterns in a manner similar to caloric restriction.
(4, 5, 34, 36, 38, 45- 47, 55, 71, 81, 99, 100)

Resveratrol and Heart Health

Resveratrol and the other polyphenols in wine are believed to account for the so-called French Paradox. The French Paradox, the fact that the rate of coronary heart disease mortality in France is lower than observed in other industrialized countries, has been attributed to an increased consumption of red wine by the French.

Resveratrol inhibits the oxidation of low-density lipoprotein (LDL) cholesterol, inhibits smooth muscle cell proliferation and inhibits platelet aggregation. Resveratrol also reduces the synthesis of lipids in the liver and inhibits the production of proatherogenic eicosanoids by human platelets and neutrophils. Thus, it helps maintain healthy levels of blood lipids and cholesterol, reduces the formation of arterial plaque and reduces the hardening and thickening of arterial walls.

It is believed that some of the beneficial effects of resveratrol are a result of its anti-oxidant properties. These include the inhibition of LDL cholesterol oxidation and the increase in nitric oxide synthesis. Nitric oxide is involved in vasodilation and improved circulation.

The inhibition of platelet aggregation translates to a reduction in the tendency to form blood clots. Resveratrol, therefore, may reduce the frequency and severity of heart attacks and strokes. It has been proposed as an alternative to low dose aspirin for this purpose. *(1, 13, 14, 18, 28, 30, 61, 62, 64, 68, 74)*

Resveratrol is an Anti-Oxidant

Resveratrol also has been found to exert a strong inhibitory effect on superoxide anion and hydrogen peroxide production by macrophages. It also has been demonstrated to decrease pro-inflammatory arachidonic acid release. It has hydroxyl-radical scavenging activity and glutathione-sparing activity. *(7, 12, 19, 20, 33, 60, 65, 94, 95)*

Cancer and Resveratrol

Resveratrol is being actively researched as both a cancer preventive and treatment. Resveratrol is a broad-spectrum agent that stops cancer in many diverse ways, including blocking estrogen and androgens and modulating genes. Cancer types that may be responsive to resveratrol include colon, neuroblastoma, esophageal, breast (all types), prostate (all types), leukemia, bone, skin, pancreas, ovarian, melanoma, liver, lung, stomach, oral, cervical, lymphoma, and thyroid.

Recent research shows that resveratrol kills cancer cells whether they do or do not have the tumor suppressor gene. It also works whether cancer cells are estrogen receptor positive or negative.

In addition to its direct anti-cancer properties, resveratrol may act as a synergist for other cancer treatments. For example, vitamin D3 converts to a steroid

82

that inhibits the growth of breast cancer cells, and researchers have found that resveratrol increases the effect of vitamin D. Other research shows that it causes drug-resistant non-Hodgkin's lymphoma cancer cells to become susceptible to certain chemotherapeutic drugs. Additional research shows that resveratrol inhibits the ability of cancer cells to metastasize, particularly to bone.

The typical western diet contains a disproportionate amount of linoleic acid. Our bodies convert a portion of our dietary linoleic acid to arachidonic acid, which is converted to hormone like substances that can promote inflammatory processes that stimulate cancer cell growth. In a study from Japan, resveratrol inhibited the growth of breast cancer cells and blocked the cancer growth promoting effects of linoleic acid. *(3, 9, 10, 24, 26, 32, 37, 40, 42, 48, 49, 58, 63, 72, 79, 89, 91)*

Alzheimer's and Resveratrol

Alzheimer's patients produce an abnormal protein known as "beta-amyloid" in their brains. Beta-amyloid provokes increased levels of free radicals and oxidative stress which damages and kills brain cells. It has been hypothesized that resveratrol can protect the brain against oxidative stress, and keep cells alive. Research shows that adding additional anti-oxidants to resveratrol provides a greater degree of protection than from resveratrol alone. Additional anti-oxidants include vitamins C and E.

Researchers have also discovered that resveratrol actually promotes the clearance of amyloid-beta molecules that have already formed. Resveratrol apparently destroys amyloid-beta by producing intracellular proteosomes that attack and dissolve the amyloid-beta plaque. Researchers have also found that resveratrol activates a gene that prolongs lifespan and that this same gene protects the brain from damage from amyloid-beta plaque. *(2, 51, 52, 54, 56, 57, 59, 75, 78, 80)*

Resveratrol Precautions

Since resveratrol is known to inhibit platelet aggregation and blood clot formation, individuals with bleeding disorders or taking anti-coagulant medications should consult their physician before using resveratrol supplements.

Other Resveratrol Considerations

It is known that most of the resveratrol taken orally is metabolized into derivative components in the digestive system and the derivative components are absorbed readily into the blood. It is also known that any resveratrol that makes it into the blood is quickly broken down to its derivative components by the liver. The question then comes, "how meaningful are those studies which measure the effects of resveratrol on cell cultures in the laboratory rather than the resveratrol derivatives that are found in the human blood?"

Some of the data referenced comes from human epidemiological studies, the observation of objective parameters such as blood tests in humans, animal studies, and studies of cell cultures in the laboratory. It may be possible that some of the positive results reported from cell culture studies may not be duplicated by oral administration in humans. Yet, the positive results epidemiological and clinical studies involving humans demonstrates that red wine polyphenols including resveratrol do have positive health benefits when consumed orally.

The literature on recent resveratrol research is massive, but does not clarify this question. Additional studies involving resveratrol derivatives will be needed to clarify this question.

Resveratrol Dosage

An obvious question is, "what dosage of resveratrol is necessary to produce an extension of human life span?" Some of the research with mice was done with a dosage of 22.4 mg per kg of body weight. That is the equivalent of 1629 mg for a 160 pound adult human. Another study yielded similar results with an equivalent dose of 124 mg per day for a 160 pound adult. Other sources claim positive results with doses of 20 mg per day for a human. Translating dosages from animals to humans is an art at best and definitive dose ranging studies are still lacking.

So, what about getting your resveratrol from natural sources, like wine? It takes approximately 41 glasses of red wine to equal the resveratrol in one 20 mg capsule. Alcohol is detrimental to health in a variety of ways especially when consumed in excess.

In addition, red wine is highly variable in resveratrol content. French farmers who demonstrated a lower incidence of heart disease consumed approximately one liter of red wine per day. At the time, it was estimated that one liter of wine contained approximately 20 mg of resveratrol. However, the wide spread use of pesticides and fungicides in vineyards has led to a drastic reduction in the resveratrol content of wine. Recall that resveratrol is produced in the grapes as a defense against damage and fungus attack. With no bugs and fungus, the grapes don't need to make resveratrol any longer. So, if you are looking for wine or grapes or growing your own, go organic and go for humid conditions that promote fungus. It is possible that grape varieties that are naturally fungus resistant may also be higher in resveratrol as well.

Chapter 21 - Green Tea

Archeological evidence suggests that tea leaves steeped in boiling water were consumed as many as 500,000 years ago. Historical evidence from China indicates that tea infusions have been used as a beverage for approximately the past 4,700 years. The cultivation of tea is believed to have begun in China or India. Today, tea is the world's most popular beverage next to water. Green tea, black tea, oolong tea, and white tea are all derived from the camellia sinensis plant and all have traditionally been consumed for their health benefits. The difference in the teas is in their processing. Green tea is made from unfermented leaves and is reputed to contain the highest concentration of polyphenols. In traditional Chinese and Ayurvedic medicine, green tea has been used as a stimulant, diuretic, astringent, and heart tonic.

Herpes and Green Tea

A number of individuals have reported in internet blogs that green tea consumption has been beneficial in reducing or controlling herpes outbreaks. At least two patents have been filed on the use of tea as a topical agent in the treatment of herpes lesions. Several reports have been published documenting the anti-viral properties of green tea constituents. *(66 - 84)*

Antiviral Properties of Green Tea

In lab tests, EGCG, found in green tea, was found to prevent HIV from attacking T-Cells. Green Tea components have been discovered to differentially inhibit the enzymes used by HIV for replication. A Chinese study found that green tea catechins could inhibit the reverse transcriptase or polymerases of several viruses including HIV-1 and Herpes Simplex-1. Various polymeric oxidation products of polyphenols have also been found to inhibit the herpes simplex virus. *(66 - 84)*

Results from several animal and human studies suggest that the polyphenols present in green tea may help treat viral hepatitis. In these studies, catechins was isolated from green tea and used in very high concentrations. It has

86

not been proven that drinking green tea confers these same benefits to people with hepatitis.

The catechins in green tea have also demonstrated activity against Influenza A and B viruses. EGCG was observed to have the highest antiviral activity but the other polyphenols also contributed to antiviral activity and the natural combination was more effective than any of the isolates. Recent studies done in Japan and China demonstrated that green tea catechins in general could inhibit the reverse transcriptase or polymerases of several types of viruses including HIV-1 and herpes simplex 1. Various polymeric oxidation products of polyphenols have also been found to inhibit the herpes simplex virus.

Tea and tea extracts have also been used as a topical treatment for herpes virus outbreaks. A patent has been filed in the UK (Number 2,293,548). Joan Hibberd, a medical doctor, found that ordinary tea works better than acyclovir as a topical treatment for herpes lesions. According to Dr Hibberd, within four or five days the lesions crust over, then disappear and do not recur for at least several months after treatment. *(1, 4, 30, 66 - 84)*

Antioxidant properties of Green Tea

The polyphenols in green tea are antioxidants. Antioxidants neutralize free radicals that can damage cells and induce genetic mutations. Free radicals contribute to the aging process and the development of cancer and heart disease. Green tea contains six primary catechin compounds: catechin, gallaogatechin, epicatechin, epigallocatechin, epicatechin gallate, and apigallocatechin gallate (EGCG). The polyphenol that has been most researched and is believed to have the most potent health benefits is EGCG. Green tea contains roughly 30% to 40% polyphenols and black tea contains only 3% to 10% polyphenols. The average cup of green tea contains about 50 to 150 mg polyphenols. *(4, 25, 59)*

Green Tea and Heart Health

Epidemiological studies indicate that the antioxidant properties of green tea may help prevent atherosclerosis, particularly coronary artery disease. Green tea lowers total cholesterol and raises HDL ("good") cholesterol in both animals and people. One epidemiological study found that men who drink green tea are more likely to have lower total cholesterol than those who do not drink green tea. Polyphenols in green tea may block the intestinal absorption of cholesterol and promote its excretion from the body. *(15, 26, 29, 33, 44, 55, 64)*

Green Tea and Cancer

Epidemiological, animal and clinical studies have demonstrated anti-cancer properties for green tea. The polyphenols in green tea are believed to play an important role in the prevention of cancer. In addition to their antioxidant properties, green tea polyphenols are believed to help kill cancer cells and stop its progression.

The types of cancers that may be favorably affected by green tea polyphenols includes bladder cancer, breast cancer, colorectal cancer, esophageal cancer, lung cancer, pancreatic cancer, prostate cancer, skin cancer, and stomach cancer. While there is evidence that green tea polyphenols may inhibit the growth of many types of cancer cells, there are enough contradictory and inconclusive results from studies to make it difficult to draw hard conclusions based on published research. Some studies show that green tea may reduce cancer rates while others suggest that it may actually increase cancer rates.
(4, 6, 7, 11 - 14, 19 - 23, 27, 28, 31, 34, 35, 37 - 40, 42, 43, 45, 46, 48, 49, 51, 53, 54, 56 - 58, 62, 65)

Green Tea and Weight Loss

Green tea extract may boost metabolism and help burn fat. This effect may be attributed to the catechins in the green tea. In addition to the polyphenols, green tea also contains alkaloids including caffeine, theobromine, and theophylline. These alkaloids provide green tea's stimulant effects. Green tea has been used traditionally to control blood sugar in the body and may help regulate glucose in the body. Animal studies suggest that green tea may help prevent the development of type 1 diabetes and slow the progression once

88

it has developed. Obesity is often associated with the development of diabetes. *(9, 64)*

Green Tea Fluoride and Aluminum

Tea, including green tea, is known to contain high concentrations of fluoride and aluminum. There is evidence that in recent times the concentration of aluminum and fluoride in tea has increased as a result of exposure to increasing air and water pollution. It appears that the tea plant has a strong tendency to concentrate aluminum and fluoride. It is likely that plant concentrations of aluminum and fluoride are highly variable depending on the soil, water, cultivation practices, and local pollution. This has not been adequately studied nor is it monitored.

Fluoride in particular is a serious political issue with proponents of fluoridation claiming that fluoride is good for us and pushing for fluoridation of drinking water, table salt, and dental products. The opponents contend that fluoride is harmful to human health and should be restricted. The proponents have the upper hand in politics and media, but a close examination of the science validates the opponents of fluoridation.

Fluoride is a chemical antagonist of iodine. Iodine is necessary for normal thyroid function. Much hypothyroidism is believed to be due, in large part, to suboptimum iodine levels. In addition, fluorosis, a disease affecting teeth and bones, especially in growing children and young adults, has been epidemiologically associated with heavy tea consumption and increased consumption of caffeinated beverages which also tend to be high in fluorides.

The element aluminum is abundant and widely distributed in nature. It is usually chemically bound in ways that make it difficult for plants to concentrate it and for the human body to absorb it. Aluminum that is absorbed into the body is believed to contribute to the development of Alzheimer's disease and renal and neurological disorders. The presence of high concentrations of fluorides makes aluminum more absorbable. Studies have shown that increased aluminum absorption is associated with tea consumption. *(86 - 100)*

Green Tea Drug Interactions

The U.S. Food and Drug Administration (FDA) includes tea on their list of "Generally Recognized as Safe" substances.

Green tea does contain caffeine and people who drink excessive amounts may experience irritability, insomnia, heart palpitation, and dizziness. Caffeine overdose can cause nausea, vomiting, diarrhea, headaches, and loss of appetite.

Some (not all) of the potential drug interactions that can occur with green tea include:

- Adenosine: The caffeine content in green tea may inhibit the hemodynamic effects of adenosine.
- Atropine: The tannin content in green tea may reduce the absorption of atropine.
- Iron supplements: The tannin content in green tea may reduce the bioavailability of iron. Green tea should be taken either 2 hours before or 4 hours following iron administration.
- Codeine: The tannin content in green tea may reduce the absorption of codeine.
- Benzodiazepines: Caffeine has been shown to reduce the sedative effects of benzodiazepines.
- Beta-blockers: Caffeine may increase blood pressure in people taking propranolol and metoprolol.
- Blood Thinning Medications: Green tea should not be taken with blood thinning medications because the herb may prevent platelets from clotting.
- Chemotherapy: Green tea may increase the effectiveness of some chemotherapy medications, specifically doxorubicin and tamoxifen. Green tea may also have an adverse effect on prostate cancer.
- Clozapine: Green tea may reduce the effectiveness of clozapine.
- Ephedrine: Green tea may increase the effects of ephedrine.
- Lithium: Green tea has been shown to reduce blood levels of lithium.
- Monoamine oxidase inhibitors: Green tea may cause a severe increase in blood pressure when taken together with MAOIs used to treat depression.

- Oral contraceptives: Oral contraceptives can prolong the amount of time caffeine stays in the body and may increase its stimulating effects.

(4, 5, 10, 17, 18, 102)

Green Tea Summary

Tea, including green tea, clearly has some good and bad characteristics. Most of the clinical and laboratory research has focused on the antioxidant polyphenols. This research has demonstrated numerous benefits including weight loss, heart health, anti-cancer effects and anti-viral effects. Its negative effects are attributed to its aluminum, fluoride, caffeine, and other stimulants.

These negative effects are too well documented to be ignored. Until there is a system created to produce tea with low fluoride and aluminum content and certify its safety, consumption of tea in all forms should probably be limited. An alternative for individuals wishing to consume the beneficial polyphenols found in green tea is to use the standardized extracts that are widely available.

Chapter 22 - Olive Leaf Extract

Olive trees are subtropical evergreen trees native to the Mediterranean region and similar climactic areas. The fruit and the oil pressed from the fruit have been used as an important food source throughout recorded history. The olive leaf has also been used as a medicine throughout recorded history.

Olive Leaf Extract Antimicrobial Properties

Research has demonstrated that olive leaf extract has antimicrobial properties that affect viruses, bacteria, fungus, yeast, and protozoa. Some of the studies were done on calcium elenolate in vitro (in the laboratory). Calcium elenolate proved highly effective in the test tube but was deactivated by blood proteins when introduced into humans. Calcium elenolate is not a natural constituent of olive leaf extract. Quoting some of this research out of context has caused some confusion in the marketing claims made for olive leaf products.

There are several polyphenols in olive leaf and olive fruit that are biologically active. Many of the polyphenols are removed from the fruit and oil during processing because they impart a bitter taste. The polyphenol most researched with respect to olive leaf extract's therapeutic properties is oleuropein. The more oleuropein in a particular product, the more effective it is likely to be. Oleuropein is metabolized into elenolic acid by the digestive process. Elenolic acid in turn has demonstrated broad spectrum antimicrobial effects.

Most of the studies quoted apply to in vitro testing. Clinical trials of olive leaf extract in the treatment of particular diseases have not been done. It is, therefore, not an approved drug or treatment for any particular disease. Nevertheless, it has been widely used as a common treatment for numerous infectious conditions supported by favorable anecdotal information.

Some viruses inhibited by olive leaf extract in vitro include rhinovirus, myxoviruses, Herpes simplex type I, Herpes simplex type II, Herpes zoster, Encephalomyocarditis,

Polio 1, 2, and 3, two strains of leukemia virus, many strains of influenza, and para- influenza viruses.

The mechanism of action of the anti-viral activity is reported to include:

- An ability to interfere with critical amino acid production essential for viruses.
- An ability to contain viral infection and/or spread by inactivating viruses or by preventing virus shedding.
- Ability to directly penetrate infected cells and stop viral replication.
- Neutralization of reverse transcriptase and protease in retroviruses.
- Stimulation of phagocytosis.

In in vitro testing, olive leaf extract has been reported to be an effective antimicrobial agent against over 50 pathogens, including Salmonella typhi, Vibrio parahaemolyticus, Staphylococcus aureus, Klebsiella pneumonia, and Escherichia col. Oleuropein has also been reported to directly stimulate macrophage activation in laboratory studies. *(13, 14, 17 - 21, 22, 35 - 40)*

Olive Leaf Extract in Protozoa Infections

Olive leaf extract has been traditionally used as a malaria treatment. Some of the old references claim that it is superior to quinine in effectiveness. *(41 - 43)*

Olive Leaf Extract in Chronic Fatigue

As an anti-fungal and anti-viral agent, olive leaf extract is currently used as a supportive agent in the management of chronic fatigue syndrome and fibromyalgia. It is hypothesized that the antimicrobial action of olive leaf extract enables it to kill infectious organisms that are believed to contribute to fatigue, low energy and chronic fatigue. There are many anecdotal reports of individuals experiencing an increase in energy and well being as a result of taking olive leaf extract.

Olive Leaf Extract and Heart Health

An olive leaf extract was reported in a laboratory study to have vasodilating effects, seemingly independent of vascular endothelial integrity. As an antioxidant oleuropein, has been reported to decrease the oxidation of LDL cholesterol and reduce the development of atherosclerosis. Olive leaf has also been reported to inhibit platelet aggregation and production of thromboxane A2, angiotensin and converting enzymes. Thus, Oleuropein has anti-clotting and anticoagulation properties.

Olive leaf extract has been reported to reduce blood pressure. One small human clinical trial has been performed with positive results. *(1 - 4, 10, 12, 27, 34)*

Olive Leaf Extract and Bone Health

French researchers have found that oleuropein, an olive leaf derived phenol stopped bone loss in an animal model of menopausal osteoporosis.

Other research has demonstrated that oleuropein has anti-inflammatory and antioxidant properties. It is believed that these properties are responsible for the reduction in bone density loss that was observed by these researchers. *(6)*

Olive Leaf Extract Precautions

Olive leaf extract will likely lower blood pressure. Therefore, anyone with hypotension or taking blood pressure lowering medications should consult their physician and use caution.

Olive leaf extract will likely lower blood sugar. Therefore, anyone with hypoglycemia or taking insulin or diabetic medications should consult their physician and use caution.

Olive leaf extract will likely reduce blood clotting. Therefore, anyone with bleeding disorders or taking anticoagulant medications should consult their physician and use caution.

Olive leaf extract may conflict with some antibiotics. Consult your physician and pharmacist before taking the two together.

Chapter 23 - Omega-3 Fatty Acids

Omega-3 fatty acids are a form of polyunsaturated fats, one of four basic types of fat that the body derives from food. Cholesterol, saturated fat, and monounsaturated fat are the others. There are several omega-3 fatty acids including alpha linolenic acid (ALA), eicosapentaenoic acid (EPA), docosahexaenoic acid (DHA) and others. The human body cannot synthesize omega-3 fatty acids but can convert alpha linolenic acid into the other omega-3 oils. Alpha linolenic acid is therefore a nutrient essential for life and is sometimes called vitamin F. Alpha linolenic acid is found in dark green leafy vegetables, flax seed oil, and certain vegetable oils. ALA from flaxseed oil is converted in the body to EPA and then DHA at an efficiency of (5%-10%), and (2%-5%) respectively. Additional sources of ALA with a high omega-3 to omega-6 ratio include chia seed oil, perilla oil, sachia inchi, purslane, lingon berry, sea buckthorn, and hemp seed oil.

Omega-3 fatty acids including eicosapentaenoic acid (EPA) and docosahexanoic acid (DHA) are found primarily in oily cold-water fish such as tuna, salmon, and mackerel. Aside from fresh seaweed, a staple of many cultures, plant foods rarely contain EPA or DHA. *(1)*

Although the body needs both omega-3 and omega-6 fatty acids to thrive, most people consume far more omega-6 fatty acids than omega 3 fatty acids. Ongoing research is consistently reporting new health benefits for the omega-3 fatty acids. Many experts now recommend consuming a better balance of these two EFAs.

Health Benefits of Omega-3 Fatty Acids

Scientists made one of the first associations between omega-3 fatty acids and human health while studying the Inuit (Eskimo) people of Greenland in the 1970s. The Inuit consumed a very high fat diet but suffered far less from coronary heart disease, rheumatoid arthritis, diabetes mellitus, and psoriasis than their European counterparts. The fat from their diet was derived from whale, seal, and salmon. Researchers eventually realized that these foods were all rich in omega-3 fatty acids, and the omega-3 fatty acids were providing real disease-countering benefits. *(2)*

Omega-3 Fatty Acids Improve Heart Health

Omega-3 fatty acids have been shown to help keep cholesterol levels low, stabilize irregular heart beat, and reduce blood pressure. Researchers now believe that alpha-linolenic acid (ALA), one of the omega-3 fats, is particularly beneficial for protecting against heart and blood vessel disease, and for lowering cholesterol and triglyceride levels. Omega-3 fatty acids are also natural blood thinners, reducing the "stickiness" of blood cells (called platelet aggregation), which can lead to such complications as blood clots and stroke. *(3 - 10)*

Omega-3 Fatty Acids Help Reduce Hypertension

Studies of large groups of people have found that the more omega-3 fatty acids people consume, the lower their overall blood pressure level is. This was the case with the Greenland Eskimos who ate a lot of oily, cold-water fish. The reduction in blood pressure is dose related. A meta-analysis of numerous trials demonstrated that 5.6 grams of fish oil per day reduced blood pressure by as much as 5.5/3.5 mm Hg. *(12 - 14)*

Omega-3 Fatty Acids Improve Autoimmune Diseases

Omega-3 fatty acids have anti-inflammatory properties. Consumption of omega-3 oils improves rheumatoid arthritis, lupus, Raynaud's disease, and other autoimmune diseases. EPA and DHA are successful at this because they can be converted into natural anti-inflammatory substances called prostaglandins and leukotrienes, compounds that help decrease inflammation and pain.

In numerous studies over the years, participants with inflammatory diseases have reported less joint stiffness, swelling, tenderness, and overall fatigue when taking omega-3 oils.

Research has shown that getting more omega-3 fatty acids enables some individuals to reduce their use of nonsteroidal anti-inflammatory drugs (NSAIDs). *(15 -19)*

Omega-3 Fatty Acids and Autism

There are currently only a few studies on the effectiveness of essential fatty acid supplementation as a treatment of autism. In one study, 18 autistic children were supplemented with fish oil for six months. Their parents described improvements in overall health, cognition, sleep patterns, social interaction, and eye contact. Another case report found that an autistic child given 540 mg of EPA per day over a four week period experienced a complete elimination of his previous anxiety about everyday events as reported by his parents and clinician. *(20 - 26)*

Omega-3 Fatty Acids Improve Depression

The brain is 60% fat and needs omega-3 fats to function properly. Now researchers have discovered a link between mood disorders and the presence of low concentrations of omega-3 fatty acids in the body. Apparently, omega-3 fats help regulate mental health problems because they enhance the ability of brain-cell receptors to comprehend mood-related signals from other neurons in the brain.

Clinical trials are underway to further investigate whether supplementing the diet with omega-3 fats will reduce the severity of such psychiatric problems as mild to moderate depression, dementia, bipolar disorder, and schizophrenia. *(21, 23)*

Omega-3 Fatty Acids Aid Cancer Prevention and Support

Preliminary research suggests that omega-3 fatty acids may help maintain healthy breast tissue and prevent breast cancer. Omega-3 fatty acids may also help prevent prostate cancer. In a recent study, participants who supplemented their diet with fish oils produced lower quantities of a carcinogen associated with colon cancer than did a placebo group. Some conflicting data suggests that Omega-3 fatty acids may stimulate the growth of metastatic colon cancer cells in the liver. More research is underway. *(41, 43 - 46)*

The Dangers of Saturated Fats and Trans Fats

Trans fats are of particular concern from a health perspective. Trans fats are fats, usually polyunsaturated oils that have been chemically hydrogenated to convert them into saturated fats. They are found in margarine and in "hydrogenated or partially hydrogenated" oils. You see this term on the majority of food labels in the supermarket. Trans fats displace healthy fats and are believed to contribute to high cholesterol, hardening of the arteries, and other health problems. *(47)*

Balancing the Ratio of Omega-3 and Omega-6 Fats

Nutritionists recognize the importance of balancing omega-3 fatty acids with omega-6 fatty acids in the diet. Because most people on a typical Western diet consume far more omega-6-rich food, the ratio is out of balance for almost everyone. The omega-6:omega-3 ratio will significantly influence the ratio of the ensuing eicosanoids (hormones), prostaglandins, leukotrienes and thromboxanes, and will alter the body's metabolic function. The ideal ratio of omega-6:omega-3 being from 3:1 to 5:1. Studies suggest that the evolutionary human diet, rich in seafood, nuts, and other sources of omega-3, may have provided such a ratio. Typical Western diets provide ratios of between 10:1 and 30:1.

This is best achieved by reducing consumption of omega-6-rich foods while increasing the intake of omega-3-rich foods. Omega-3 rich foods include: Atlantic salmon and other fatty, preferably cold-water fish, including herring, sardines, Atlantic halibut, bluefish, tuna, and Atlantic mackerel. Another good source of Omega-3 fats is wild game, including venison, and buffalo. The best sources of alpha linoleic acid, ALA, are flaxseed oil, chia oil, kiwi oil, perilla oil, purslane, lingon berry, and sea buckthorn. ALA is the plant derived oil that is the precursor of EPA and DHA.

Omega-6 oils are derived from safflower, sunflower, corn, soya, evening primrose, pumpkin seeds, and wheat

germ. These are the oils that we generally need less of. Remember, however, that some Omega-6 oils are essential for optimum health.
(27 - 31)

Cautions and Contraindications for Omega-3 Oils

Omega-3 oils can reduce blood clotting and act as a blood thinner. If you are taking anti-coagulant drugs, have a bleeding disorder, or are being treated for a medical condition, you should consult your physician before using Omega-3 supplements. Blood tests that measure clotting time can be used to ensure these nutrients are not reducing the clotting factors in your blood to abnormal levels.

The maximum safe daily dosage recommended by the United States Food and Drug Administration for a 70-kg human is a total of 3 g/day intake of EPA and DHA omega-3 fatty acids from conventional and dietary sources.

Anti-viral properties of fatty acids

Research has demonstrated that unsaturated free fatty acids such as oleic, arachidonic, or linoleic at concentrations of 5–25 µg/ml inactivate enveloped viruses such as herpes, influenza, Sendai, and Sindbis within minutes of contact. At these concentrations the fatty acids are innocuous to animal host cells in vitro.

Naked viruses, such as polio, SV40, or EMC are not affected by these fatty acids. US Patent 4,841,023 applies to the inactivation of viruses in blood plasma. According to the patent claims, unsaturated fatty acids with at least one double bond in the CIS configuration and containing 16 to 20 carbon atoms are effective. The list includes 11-eicosenoic acid, arachidonic acid, linoleic acid, linolenic acid, palmitoleic acid, elaidic acid, linolenic acid, gamma-linolenic acid, palmitic acid, and arachidic acid.

Research has shown that short-chain and long-chain saturated fatty acids have no or a very small anti-viral effect at the highest concentrations tested. Medium-chain saturated and long-chain unsaturated fatty acids, on the other hand, were all highly active against the enveloped viruses. The loss

100

of infectivity was attributed to a disruption of the lipoprotein envelope of these virons, as observed in an electron microscope.   Lauric and Caprylic acid (from coconut oil) was shown to be the most effective at inactivating viruses. *(33, 48, 49)*

Appendix A

The Lysine to Arginine Ratio in Foods

Transcribed and calculated using data from the *Agricultural Handbook, 1-23, U.S. Department of Agriculture*. Lysine to arginine ratio.

The higher the food on the list, the better for preventing herpes. Foods toward the bottom of the list favor herpes outbreaks, while those at the top of the list discourage outbreaks.

	Weight (gm)	Lys (mg)	Arg (mg)	Ratio ys/Arg
Plain Yogurt	227	706	237	2.979
Fruit Yogurt, lowfat	227	810	272	2.978
Plain Yogurt, skim	227	1160	391	2.967
Plain Yogurt, lowfat	227	1060	359	2.953
Swiss Cheese	28	733	263	2.787
Gruyere Cheese	28	768	276	2.783
Edam Cheese	28	754	273	2.762
American Cheese Spread	28	427	155	2.755
Gouda Cheese	28	752	273	2.755
Whey, dry, sweet	7.5	77	28	2.750
Blue Cheese	28	526	202	2.604
Provolone Cheese	28	750	290	2.586
Papaya	454	76	30	2.533
Brie Cheese	28	525	208	2.524
Camembert Cheese	28	501	199	2.518
Parmesan Cheese	28	937	373	2.512
Parmesan Cheese, grated	5	192	77	2.494
Gjetost Cheese	28	231	93	2.484
Goat Milk	244	708	291	2.433
Brick Cheese	28	602	248	2.427
Muenster Cheese	28	606	250	2.424
Beets	136	72	30	2.400
Limburger Cheese	28	475	198	2.399
Tilsit Cheese	28	578	241	2.398
Port du salut Cheese	28	563	235	2.396
Processed Swiss Cheese	28	696	293	2.375
Cream Cheese	28	192	81	2.370
Mozzarella Cheese, parts	28	699	295	2.369
Processed American Cheese	28	623	263	2.369
Mozzarella Cheese	28	559	236	2.369
Neufchatel Cheese	28	253	107	2.364
Butter	14.1	9	4	2.250
Colby Cheese	28	561	254	2.209
Monterey Jack Cheese	28	578	262	2.206

	Weight (gm)	Lys (mg)	Arg (mg)	Ratio Lys/Arg
Cheshire Cheese	28	551	250	2.204
Cheddar Cheese	28	588	267	2.202
Buttermilk	245	679	309	2.197
Skim Milk	245	663	302	2.195
Half and Half Cream	242	568	259	2.193
Sherbet	193	171	78	2.192
Condensed Milk, sweetened	306	1920	876	2.192
Chocolate Milk	250	629	287	2.192
Nonfat Milk, dry	120	3440	1570	2.191
Lowfat Milk, 2%	244	644	294	2.190
Evaporated Milk	126	681	311	2.190
Ice Cream	133	381	174	2.190
Whole Milk	244	637	291	2.189
Whole Milk, dry	128	2670	1220	2.189
Nonfat Milk, dry, instant	68	1890	864	2.188
Ice Milk	131	409	187	2.187
Whipping Cream, heavy	238	387	177	2.186
Evaporated Milk, skim	128	763	349	2.186
Whipping Cream, light	239	411	188	2.186
Ice Cream, rich	148	327	150	2.180
Mango	300	85	39	2.179
Whipped Cream, pressurize	60	152	70	2.171
Apricot	114	103	48	2.146
Coffee Cream	15	32	15	2.133
Apple	150	17	8	2.125
Ricotta Cheese	246	3290	1550	2.123
Ricotta Cheese, part skim	246	3320	1570	2.115
Pear, dried	175	116	56	2.071
Eggnog	254	758	378	2.005
Applesauce, unsweetened	244	24	12	2.000
Crabapple, slices	110	28	14	2.000
Loquat	16	2	1	2.000
Apple, dried	64	37	19	1.947
Pear	180	23	12	1.917
Apricot, dried	35	89	49	1.816
Cottage Cheese, creamed	210	2120	1190	1.782
Cottage Cheese, Lowfat 2%	226	2510	1410	1.780
Cottage Cheese, dry	145	2020	1140	1.772
Fig, dried	189	228	131	1.740
Fig	65	19	11	1.727
Human Milk	246	168	105	1.600
Avocado	272	189	119	1.588
Salmon	85	1550	1000	1.550
Swordfish	85	1550	1000	1.550
Haddock	85	1480	961	1.540
Smelt	85	1380	897	1.538
Snapper	85	1600	1040	1.538
Pollock	85	1520	989	1.537
Eel	85	1440	938	1.535
Catfish	85	1420	925	1.535
Anchovy, in oil, drained	20	531	346	1.535

	Weight (gm)	Lys (mg)	Arg (mg)	Ratio Lys/Arg
Whitefish	85	1490	971	1.535
Tuna, in water	165	4480	2920	1.534
Cod	85	1390	906	1.534
Flat fish, flounder and s	85	1470	959	1.533
Mackerel	85	1450	946	1.533
Shark	85	1640	1070	1.533
Carp	85	1390	907	1.533
Pike	85	1500	979	1.532
Herring	85	1400	914	1.532
Sardines, in oil, drained	24	542	354	1.531
Bass	85	1380	902	1.530
Perch	85	1450	948	1.530
Bluefish	85	1560	1020	1.529
Halibut	85	1620	1060	1.528
Tomato	123	41	27	1.519
Turnips	130	47	31	1.516
Tomato juice	243	54	36	1.500
Soybean sprouts	70	386	266	1.451
Canadian Style Bacon	454	7370	5100	1.445
Wild pheasant	371	7470	5240	1.426
Pork Spareribs	454	4730	3340	1.416
Tomato paste	262	282	200	1.410
Liver cheese	28	334	237	1.409
Chicken, dark meat, w/o s	109	1860	1320	1.409
Chicken, light meat w/o s	88	1730	1230	1.407
Chicken neck	79	298	212	1.406
Summer sausage	23	318	228	1.395
Pineapple	155	39	28	1.393
Pork leg	454	7550	5530	1.365
Pork loin chop	151	1950	1430	1.364
Pork Shoulder	454	7140	5240	1.363
Potato	150	190	140	1.357
Chicken breast	181	2500	1870	1.337
Cream of Mushroom soup	244	127	95	1.337
Turkey noodle soup	244	212	159	1.333
Celery	120	32	24	1.333
Chicken drumstick	110	1160	872	1.330
Potato, baking	202	283	214	1.322
Beef Flank steak	454	7270	5500	1.322
Chicken gumbo	244	161	122	1.320
Chicken noodle soup	241	219	166	1.319
Beef Round steak	454	7320	5550	1.319
Beef noodle soup	244	261	198	1.318
Vegetable w/beef soup	244	344	261	1.318
Cream of Asparagus soup	244	112	85	1.318
Porterhouse steak	454	6560	4980	1.317
Beef T-bone steak	454	6330	4810	1.316
Beef Sirloin steak	454	6880	5230	1.315
Knockwurst	68	634	482	1.315
Beef Rib roast	454	6050	4600	1.315
Beef Short ribs	454	5430	4130	1.315

	Weight (gm)	Lys (mg)	Arg (mg)	Ratio Lys/Arg
Beef Chuck roast	454	6900	5250	1.314
Beef Tenderloin	454	6990	5320	1.314
Persimmon	200	55	42	1.310
Squash, summer	130	85	65	1.308
Chicken leg	231	2470	1890	1.307
Chicken, light meat	116	1920	1470	1.306
Ham, boneless	454	6750	5170	1.306
Chicken canned, boned	142	2500	1920	1.302
Turkey, dark meat	152	2620	2020	1.297
Cream of chicken soup	244	215	166	1.295
Chicken heart	6.1	79	61	1.295
Turkey, light meat	180	3540	2740	1.292
Bratwurst, ckd	85	910	706	1.289
Turkey, canned boned	142	3040	2360	1.288
Italian sausage, ckd	67	1020	792	1.288
Pork sausage	28	252	196	1.286
Wild quail	405	6660	5180	1.286
Chicken thigh	120	1310	1020	1.284
Chicken, dark meat	160	2150	1680	1.280
Goose, domesticated	320	4010	3150	1.273
Pork and beef sausage	13	141	111	1.270
Bologna, beef and pork	28	250	198	1.263
Peach, dried	130	151	120	1.258
Black bean soup	247	415	331	1.254
Bean w/ frankfurters soup	250	415	331	1.254
Peach	115	20	16	1.250
Corned Beef, brisket	454	5100	4100	1.244
Pastrami	28	375	302	1.242
Bologna, beef	28	254	205	1.239
Frankfurter, beef	45	389	314	1.239
Ground beef, regular	113	1560	1260	1.238
Cream of celery soup	244	73	59	1.237
Ground beef, lean	113	1670	1350	1.237
Chicken liver	32	35	352	1.236
Duck liver	44	624	505	1.236
Turkey liver	102	1540	1250	1.232
Mortadella	28	358	291	1.230
Goose liver	94	1160	943	1.230
Plum	5.5	90	74	1.216
Green beans	110	97	80	1.213
Chicken back	177	1090	900	1.211
Beef smoked, chopped	28	467	386	1.210
Pork Bacon	454	2900	2400	1.208
Beef, dried	28	673	557	1.208
Brotwurst	28	323	268	1.205
Polish sausage	28	315	262	1.202
Salami, hard	10	182	152	1.197
Bologna, pork	28	341	285	1.196
Chicken wing	90	698	585	1.193
Braunschweiger	28	258	217	1.189

	Weight (gm)	Lys (mg)	Arg (mg)	Ratio Lys/Arg
Duck, domesticated	287	2610	2210	1.181
Lentil sprouts	77	548	470	1.166
Lettuce, romaine	56	58	50	1.160
Lettuce, iceberg	75	60	52	1.154
Caviar, black and red	16	293	254	1.154
Cauliflower	100	108	96	1.125
Vienna sausage	16	127	113	1.124
Liver	113	1570	1420	1.106
Guava	112	21	19	1.105
New England Clam Chowder	244	251	229	1.096
Cream of potato soup	244	83	76	1.092
Spinach	55	98	90	1.089
Kale	67	132	123	1.073
Chicken rice soup	241	251	234	1.073
Kielbasa	28	286	267	1.071
Frankfurter, beef and por	45	407	382	1.065
Whole Egg	50	410	388	1.057
Egg White	33	206	195	1.056
Whole Egg, dried	5	155	147	1.054
Watermelon	160	99	94	1.053
Cabbage, Chinese	70	62	59	1.051
Corn	154	210	200	1.050
Sweet potato	130	105	100	1.050
Turnip greens	55	54	52	1.038
Abalone	85	1090	1060	1.028
Oysters	84	444	433	1.025
Clams	180	1720	1680	1.024
Scallops	85	1060	1040	1.019
Banana	175	55	54	1.019
Asparagus	134	194	192	1.010
Oat flakes	48	583	579	1.007
Mayonnaise	185	1400	1400	1.000
Vegetarian vegetable soup	241	99	99	1.000
Beet greens	38	20	20	1.000
Endive	50	32	32	1.000
Leeks	124	97	97	1.000
Pumpkin	245	96	96	1.000
Shrimp	85	1500	1510	0.993
Crab	85	1350	1360	0.993
Pea soup w/ham	253	696	703	0.990
Lima beans, cooked	170	765	775	0.987
Egg Yolk	17	189	193	0.979
Okra	100	82	84	0.976
Broccoli	88	124	128	0.969
Chicken gizzard	37	465	484	0.961
Strawberries	149	37	39	0.949
Collards	186	140	72	0.931
Minestrone soup	241	183	198	0.924
Carrots	110	44	48	0.917
Dates	83	50	55	0.909
Peppers, sweet	100	38	42	0.905

106

	Weight (gm)	Lys (mg)	Arg (mg)	Ratio Lys/Arg
Radish	45	16	18	0.889
Watercress	104	172	200	0.860
Swiss chard	36	36	42	0.857
Eggplant	82	42	50	0.840
Tomato soup	244	51	61	0.836
Cabbage, common	70	40	48	0.833
Wheat germ	180	1330	1790	0.743
Peas, green	146	463	625	0.741
Brussels sprouts	88	130	178	0.730
Tangerine	116	27	37	0.730
Orange	180	62	85	0.729
Onions, green	100	4	6	0.667
Mushrooms	70	48	72	0.667
Cucumber	104	22	36	0.611
Wheat granules	28.4	101	169	0.598
Corn grits	242	68	114	0.596
Snails	85	1250	2100	0.595
Wheat, shredded	23.6	79	133	0.594
Wheat flakes	33	101	171	0.591
Cream of wheat	251	98	166	0.590
Pistachios, shelled	128	1640	2790	0.588
Corn, puffed	28.4	65	112	0.580
Wheat, puffed	12	49	85	0.576
Squash, winter	205	902	1590	0.567
Bran flakes	47	177	314	0.564
Elderberries	145	38	68	0.559
Plantain	148	89	160	0.556
Oats, puffed	28.4	175	320	0.547
Oatmeal	234	78	147	0.531
Cashews	160	246	470	0.523
Chestnuts, fresh	160	246	470	0.523
Rice, puffed	14	38	73	0.521
Yams	200	89	191	0.466
Pumpkin seeds & squash	140	2530	5570	0.454
Garlic	3	8	19	0.421
Macadamia nuts	134	434	1200	0.362
Blackberries	145	17	49	0.347
Blueberries	145	17	49	0.347
Onions, mature	160	90	262	0.344
Grapes, slip skin	153	13	42	0.310
Grapes, adherent skin	160	24	78	0.308
Peanuts	144	1450	5050	0.287
Peanut butter	15	176	613	0.287
Coconut, shredded	80	118	437	0.270
Almonds	142	946	3540	0.267
Rutabaga	140	55	207	0.266
Pecans	108	315	1190	0.265
Sesame seeds	150	1240	4990	0.248
Hickory nuts	15	70	298	0.235
Brazil nuts	140	757	3350	0.226
Tahini	15	82	378	0.217

	Weight (gm)	Lys (mg)	Arg (mg)	Ratio Lys/Arg
Grape juice	253	25	119	0.210
Tangerine juice	247	17	84	0.202
Pine nuts	28	256	1330	0.192
Orange juice	248	22	117	0.188
Hazelnuts	135	459	2480	0.185
Walnuts	100	466	2520	0.185

Appendix B - Patents related to Natural Herpes Treatments

Over the years, various substances have been postulated as medications for the various kinds of herpes.

Examples include:

- A mixture of vitamin C and vitamin P for herpes simplex labialis (U.S. Pat. No. 4,049,798),

- A mixture of kelp and a carrier (U.S. Pat. No. 4,117,120),

- Extract of mountain ash berries (U.S. Pat. No. 4,132,782),

- A water soluble extract from marine red algae (U.S. Pat. No. 4,162,308),

- An antiviral lignosulfate (U.S. Pat. No. 4,185,097),

- 1-amino-2, 4-ethanobicyclo[3, 3, 1]nonane or salts thereof (U.S. Pat. No. 4,230,725),

- A suspension of boric acid, tannic acid, and salicylic acid, preferably in an ethanol solvent/carrier (U.S. Pat. No. 4,285,934).

Appendix C - Links to Herpes Related Blogs

In an atmosphere where sanctioned scientific and medical data are lacking, and sales claims may be suspect, there is another possible source of information. That is: Reports by honest individuals posted on the internet. Such reports and such individuals do exist.

Use your search engine to look for blogs related to herpes and specific treatment topics. Listed here are a few that this author located on a quick search.

http://bht-coldsores.blogspot.com/

http://curezone.org/forums/fm.asp?i=1089079

http://www.herpes-coldsores.com/messageforum/showthread.php?s=4bdb5937305b4d8a1b0dcda3e63f49c2&t=2970&page=2

References

References - Chapter 1 - Herpes Virus Overview

(1) http://www.cdc.gov/ncidod/diseases/ebv.htm

(2) Ryan KJ, Ray CG (editors) (2004). *Sherris Medical Microbiology*, 4th ed., McGraw Hill, pp. 556; 566–9.

(3) Human Herpesvirus-6 Infection in Children - A Prospective Study of Complications and Reactivation, Hall et al... N Engl J Med. 1994 Aug 18;331(7):432-8.

(4) http://www.blackwell-synergy.com/servlet/useragent?func=synergy&&synergyAction=showAbstract&doi=10.1034/j.1600-0404.2002.1o050.x, Acta Neurol Scand.

(5) Komaroff AL. (2006 Dec). "Is human herpesvirus-6 a trigger for chronic fatigue syndrome". *J Clin Virol.* 37 (Suppl 1): S39-46.

(6) http://www.wisconsinlab.com/hiv.htm, Wisconsin Viral Research Group

(7) Fotheringham J, Donati D, Akhyani N, Fogdell-Hahn A, Vortmeyer A, Heiss JD, Williams E, Weinstein S, Bruce DA, Gaillard WD, Sato S, Theodore WH, Jacobson S (2007). "Association of human herpesvirus-6B with mesial temporal lobe epilepsy." *PLoS Med.* 4 (5): e180.

(8) http://www.cdc.gov/ncidod/eid/vol5no3/campadelli.htm

(9) http://www.cdc.gov/ncidod/eid/vol10no8/03-0788.htm

(10) http://en.wikipedia.org/wiki/Kaposi%27s_sarcoma-associated_herpesvirus

(11) American Social Health Association. Sexually Transmitted Diseases in America: How Many Cases and at What Cost? Menlo Park, CA: Kaiser Family Foundation, 1998.

(12) Fleming DT, *et al*. Herpes Simplex Virus type 2 in the United States, 1976 to 1994. *NEJM* 1997; 337:1105-11.

(13) Institute of Medicine. Committee on Prevention and Control of Sexually Transmitted Diseases. *The Hidden Epidemic: Confronting Sexually Transmitted Diseases*. Eng TR and Butler WT, eds. Washington, DC: National Academy Press, 1997.

(14) National Center for Health Statistics (US) http://www.cdc.gov/nchs/

(15) National Statistics Online (UK) http://www.satistics.gov.uk/

(16) Statistics Canada: the national statistical agency providing (Canada) http://www.statcan.ca

(17) Fujie Xu, MD, PhD; Maya R. Sternberg, PhD; Benny J. Kottiri, PhD; Geraldine M. McQuillan, PhD; Francis K. Lee, PhD; Andre J. Nahmias, MD; Stuart M. Berman, MD, ScM; Lauri E. Markowitz, MD; *Journal of the American Medical Association,* August 23/30, 2006.

Chapter 6 - Vitamin A References

(1) Mostad SB, Kreiss JK, et al. Cervical shedding of herpes simplex virus in human immunodeficiency virus-infected women: effects of hormonal contraception, pregnancy, and vitamin A deficiency. *J Infect Dis* . 2000 Jan;181(1):58-63.

(2) Pomponi F, Cariati R, et al. Retinoids irreversibly inhibit in vitro growth of Epstein-Barr virus-immortalized B lymphocytes. *Blood*. 1996 Oct 15;88(8):3147-59.

(3) Santos MS, Meydani SN, et al. Natural killer cell activity in elderly men is enhanced by beta-carotene supplementation. *Am J Clin Nutr.* 1996 Nov;64(5)772-7.

(4) http://www.lef.org/protocols/infections/herpes_shingles_01.htm

(5) Semba RD. Vitamin A, immunity, and infection. *Clin Infect Dis* 1994;19:489–99 [review].

(6) Glasziou PP, Mackerras DEM. Vitamin A supplementation in infectious diseases: a meta-analysis. *BMJ* 1993;306:366–70.

(7) Penn ND, Purkins L, Kelleher J, et al. The effect of dietary supplementation with vitamins A, C and E on cell-mediated immune function in elderly long-stay patients: a randomized controlled trial. *Age Ageing* 1991;20:169–74.

(8) de la Fuente M, Ferrandez MD, Burgos MS, et al. Immune function in aged women is improved by ingestion of vitamins C and E. *Can J Physiol Pharmacol* 1998;76:373–80.

(9) Semba RD. Impact of vitamin A on immunity and infection in developing countries. In: Bendich A, Decklebaum RJ, eds. Preventive Nutrition: The Comprehensive Guide for Health Professionals. 2nd ed. Totowa: Humana Press Inc; 2001:329-346.

(10) McCullough, F. et al. The effect of vitamin A on epithelial integrity. Proceedings of the Nutrition Society. 1999; volume 58: pages 289-293.

(11) Semba RD. The role of vitamin A and related retinoids in immune function. Nutr Rev. 1998;56(1 Pt 2):S38-48.

(12) http://lpi.oregonstate.edu/infocenter/vitamins/vitaminA/

(13) Rothman KJ, Moore LL, Singer MR, et al. Teratogenicity of high vitamin A intake. *N Engl J Med* 1995;333:1369–73.

112

(14) Mastroiacovo P, Mazzone T, Addis A, et al. High vitamin A intake in early pregnancy and major malformations: a multicenter prospective controlled study. *Teratology* 1999;59:7–11.

(15) Biesalski HK. Comparative assessment of the toxicology of vitamin A and retinoids in man. *Toxicology* 1989;57:117–61.

(16) Azais-Braesco V, Pascal G. Vitamin A in pregnancy: requirements and safety limits. *Am J Clin Nutr* 2000;71(5 Suppl):1325S–33S [review].

(17) Wiegand UW, Hartmann S, Hummler H. Safety of vitamin A: recent results. *Int J Vitam Nutr Res* 1998;68:411–6 [review].

(18) Myhre, et al., "Water-miscible, emulsified, and solid forms of retinol supplements are more toxic than oil-based preparations," *Am J Clin Nutr*, 78 (2003) 1152-9.

(19) http://www.emedicine.com/emerg/topic638.htm

(20) http://www.emedicine.com/med/topic2382.htm

(21) Sale TA, Stratman E (2004). "Carotenemia associated with green bean ingestion." *Pediatr Dermatol* 21 (6): 657–9.

(22) Nishimura Y, Ishii N, Sugita Y, Nakajima H (1998). "A case of carotenodermia caused by a diet of the dried seaweed called Nori." *J. Dermatol.* 25 (10): 685–7.

(23) Takita Y, Ichimiya M, Hamamoto Y, Muto M (2006). "A case of carotenemia associated with ingestion of nutrient supplements." *J. Dermatol.* 33 (2): 132–4.

(24) http://aje.oxfordjournals.org/cgi/gca?allch=&SEARCHID=1&FULLTEXT=forsmo&FIRSTINDEX=0&hits=10&RESULTFORMAT=&gca=amjepid%3Bkwm320v1

(25) Gerald Litwack, *Vitamin A.* (Vitamins and Hormones. Vol. 75.) 412 pp., illustrated. San Diego, CA, Elsevier Academic Press, 2007. ISBN 978-0-12-709875-3.

Chapter 7 - Vitamin C References

(1) De Souza MC, Walker AF, et al. A synergistic effect of a daily supplement for 1 month of 200 mg magnesium plus 50 mg vitamin B6 for the relief of anxiety-related premenstrual symptoms: a randomized, double-blind, crossover study. *J Womens Health Gend Based Med.* 2000 Mar;9(2):131-9.

(2) Terezhalmy GT, Bottomley WK, et al. The use of water-soluble bioflavonoid-ascorbic acid complex in the treatment of recurrent herpes labialis. *Oral Surg Oral Med Oral Pathol.* 1978 Jan;45(1):56-62.

(3) Hovi T, Hirvimies A, et al. Topical treatment of recurrent mucocutaneous herpes with ascorbic acid-containing solution. *Antiviral Res.* 1995 Jun;27(3):263-70.

(4) Higdon, Jane, Ph.D. (2006-01-31). Vitamin C. Oregon State University, Micronutrient Information Center.

(5) Levine M, Rumsey SC, Wang Y, Park JB, Daruwala R. Vitamin C. In Stipanuk MH (ed): "Biochemical and Physiological Aspects of Human Nutrition." Philadelphia: W B Saunders, pp 541–567, 2000.

(6) Prockop DJ, Kivirikko KI: Collagens: molecular biology, diseases, and potentials for therapy. Annu Rev Biochem 64:403–434, 1995.

(7) Peterkofsky B: Ascorbate requirement for hydroxylation and secretion of procollagen: relationship to inhibition of collagen synthesis in scurvy. Am J Clin Nutr 54:1135S–1140S, 1991.

(8) Kivirikko KI, Myllyla R: Post-translational processing of procollagens. Ann N Y Acad Sci 460:187–201, 1985.

(9) McGee, William, M.D., M.H.A., Assistant Professor of Medicine and Surgery, Tufts University School of Medicine; Medical Encyclopedia: Ascorbic acid.

(10) Rebouche CJ (1991). "Ascorbic acid and carnitine biosynthesis." *Am J Clin Nutr* 54 (6 Suppl): 1147S-1152S.

(11) Dunn WA, Rettura G, Seifter E, Englard S (1984). "Carnitine biosynthesis from gamma-butyrobetaine and from exogenous protein-bound 6-N-trimethyl-L-lysine by the perfused guinea pig liver. Effect of ascorbate deficiency on the in situ activity of gamma-butyrobetaine hydroxylase." *J Biol Chem* 259 (17): 10764-70.

(12) Levine M, Dhariwal KR, Washko P, Welch R, Wang YH, Cantilena CC, Yu R: Ascorbic acid and reaction kinetics in situ: a new approach to vitamin requirements. J Nutr Sci Vitaminol (Tokyo) Spec No:169–172, 1992.

(13) Kaufman S: Dopamine-beta-hydroxylase. J Psychiatr Res 11: 303–316, 1974.

(14) Eipper BA, Milgram SL, Husten EJ, Yun HY, Mains RE: Peptidylglycine alpha-amidating monooxygenase: a multifunctional protein with catalytic, processing, and routing domains. Protein Sci 2:489–497, 1993.

(16) Eipper BA, Stoffers DA, Mains RE: The biosynthesis of neuropeptides: peptide alpha-amidation. Annu Rev Neurosci 15:57–85, 1992.

(17) Englard S, Seifter S (1986). "The biochemical functions of ascorbic acid." *Annu. Rev. Nutr.* 6: 365-406.

(18) Lindblad B, Lindstedt G, Lindstedt S: The mechanism of enzymic formation of homogentisate from p-hydroxyphenylpyruvate. J Am Chem Soc 92:7446–7449, 1970.

114

(19) C Matthias A. Hediger , *Nature Medicine* 8, 445 - 446 (2002) doi:10.1038/nm0502-445.

(20) Jariwalla, Raxit and Harakeh, Steve. Antiviral and immunomodulatory activities of ascorbic acid. In Subcellular Biochemistry, Volume 25: Ascorbic Acid: Biochemistry and Biomedical Cell Biology, edited by J. Robin Harris, NY: Plenum Press, pp. 215-231 (1996).

(21) http://www.iom.edu/Object.File/Master/7/296/webtablevitamins.pdf

(22) Milton K (2003). "Micronutrient intakes of wild primates: are humans different?" *Comp Biochem Physiol A Mol Integr Physiol* 136 (1): 47-59.

(23) Pauling, Linus. "Evolution and the need for ascorbic acid." *Proc Natl Acad Sci U S A* 67 (4): 1643-8.

(24) Stone, Irwin (1972). The Healing Factor: Vitamin C Against Disease. Grosset and Dunlap. ISBN 0-448-11693-6.

(25) http://www.seanet.com/~alexs/ascorbate/197x/stone-i-orthomol_psych-1979-v8-n2-p58.htm

(26) http://www.orthomed.com/klenner.htm

(27) Pauling L (1970). "Evolution and the need for ascorbic acid." *Proc. Natl. Acad. Sci. U.S.A.* 67 (4): 1643-8.

(28) Stone, Irwin. Homo sapiens ascorbicus, a biochemically corrected robust human mutant. Med. Hypotheses 5: 711-722, 1979.

(29) Harakeh S, Jariwalla R, Pauling L (1990). "Suppression of human immunodeficiency virus replication by ascorbate in chronically and acutely infected cells." *Proc Natl Acad Sci U S A* 87 (18): 7245-9.

(30) http://www.physorg.com/news87833644.html

(31) Dawson E, Evans D, Harris W, Teter M, McGanity W (1999). "The effect of ascorbic acid supplementation on the blood lead levels of smokers." *J Am Coll Nutr* 18 (2): 166-70.

(32) Simon JA, Hudes ES (1999). "Relationship of ascorbic acid to blood lead levels." *JAMA* 281 (24): 2289-93.

(33) http://lpi.oregonstate.edu/f-w99/kidneystones.html

(34) http://lpi.oregonstate.edu/s-s00/arteries.html

(35) http://lpi.oregonstate.edu/f-w01/cancer.html

(36) http://lpi.oregonstate.edu/f-w98/genetic.html

(37) Orient, Jane M.D., Treating Herpes Zoster with Vitamin C: Two Case Reports, J. Am. Phys. Surg., Spring 2006.

115

(38) Boyd, Herschell H., Treatment of Iritis and Herpes Zoster with Vitamin C, Journal of Orthomolecular Medicine Vol. 10, No. 2, 1995.

(39) Yokoo S, Furumoto K, Hiyama E, Miwa N. Slow-down of age-dependent telomere shortening is executed in human skin keratinocytes by hormesis-like-effects of trace hydrogen peroxide or by anti-oxidative effects of pro-vitamin C in common concurrently with reduction of intracellular oxidative stress. J Cell Biochem. 2004 Oct 15;93(3):588-97.

(40) Wintergerst ES, Maggini S, Hornig DH. Immune-enhancing role of vitamin C and zinc and effect on clinical conditions. Ann Nutr Metab. 2006;50(2):85-94.

(41) Gorton HC, Jarvis K. The effectiveness of vitamin C in preventing and relieving the symptoms of virus-induced respiratory infections. J Manipulative Physiol Ther. 1999 Oct;22(8):530-3.

(42) Hemila H, Douglas RM. Vitamin C and acute respiratory infections. Int J Tuberc Lung Dis. 1999 Sep;3(9):756-61.

(43) Harakeh S, Jariwalla RJ. Comparative study of the anti-HIV activities of ascorbate and thiol-containing reducing agents in chronically HIV-infected cells. Am J Clin Nutr. 1991 Dec;54(6 Suppl):1231S-5S.

(44) Muller F, Svardal AM, Nordoy I, et al. Virological and immunological effects of antioxidant treatment in patients with HIV infection. Eur J Clin Invest. 2000 Oct;30(10):905-14.

(45) Rivas CI, Vera JC, Guaiquil VH, et al. Increased uptake and accumulation of vitamin C in human immunodeficiency virus 1-infected hematopoietic cell lines. J Biol Chem. 1997 Feb 28;272(9):5814-20.

(46) Gaby AR. Natural remedies for Herpes simplex. Altern Med Rev. 2006 Jun;11(2):93-101.

(47) Zureick M. Treatment of singles and herpes with vitamin C intravenously. I Des Practiciens. 1950;(64):585.

(48) Hovi T, Hirvimies A, Stenvik M, et al. Topical treatment of recurrent mucocutaneous herpes with ascorbic acid-containing solution. Antiviral Res. 1995 Jun;27(3):263-70.

(49) Cinatl J, Cinatl J, Weber B, et al. In vitro inhibition of human cytomegalovirus replication in human foreskin fibroblasts and endothelial cells by ascorbic acid 2-phosphate. Antiviral Res. 1995 Aug;27(4):405-18.

Chapter 8 - Zinc References

(1) Hershfinkel Michal, Silverman William F, and Sekler Israel (2007). "The Zinc Sensing Receptor, a Link Between Zinc and Cell Signaling". *Mol Med* 13 (7-8): 331-336.

(2) King JC, Cousins RJ. Zinc. In: Shils ME, Shike M, Ross AC, Caballero B, Cousins RJ, eds. Modern Nutrition in Health and Disease. 10th ed. Baltimore: Lippincott Williams & Wilkins; 2006:271-285.

(3) Hambidge M. Human zinc deficiency. J Nutr. 2000;130(5S Suppl):1344S-1349S.

(4) Shankar AH and Prasad AS. Zinc and immune function: The biological basis of altered resistance to infection. Am J Clin Nutr. 1998;68:447S-463S.

(5) Beck FW, Prasad AS, Kaplan J, Fitzgerald JT, Brewer GJ. Changes in cytokine production and T cell subpopulations in experimentally induced zinc-deficient humans. Am J Physiol 1997;272:E1002-1007.

(6) Shankar, A.H. & Prasad, A.S. Zinc and immune function: the biological basis of altered resistance to infection. American Journal of Clinical Nutrition. 1998; volume 68: pages 447S-463S.

(7) Shambaugh GE Jr. Zinc: the neglected nutrient. Am J Otol 1989 Mar;10(2):156-60.

(8) Cuevas LE, Koyanagi A. Zinc and infection: a review. Ann Trop Paediatr . 2005 Sep;25(3):149-60.

(9) Godfrey HR, Godfrey NJ, et al. A randomized clinical trial on the treatment of oral herpes with topical zinc oxide/glycine. Altern Ther Health Med . 2001 May-Jun;7(3):49-56.

(10) Chandra RK. Effect of vitamin and trace-element supplementation on immune responses and infection in elderly subjects. Lancet. 1992 Nov 7;340(8828):1124-7.

(11) Girodon F, Lombard M, et al. Effect of micronutrient supplementation on infection in institutionalized elderly subjects: a controlled trial. Ann Nutr Metab. 1997;41(2):98-107.

(12) Arens M, Travis S. Zinc salts inactivate clinical isolates of herpes simplex virus in-vitro. J Clin Microbiol 2000;38:1758–62.

(13) Wahba A. Topical application of zinc solutions: A new treatment for herpes simplex infections of the skin? Acta Derm Venereol 1980;60:175–7.

(14) Finnerty EF. Topical zinc in the treatment of herpes simplex. Cutis 1986;37:130–1.

(15) Brody I. Topical treatment of recurrent herpes simplex and post-herpetic erythema multiforme with low concentrations of zinc sulphate solution. Br J Derm 1981;104:191–4.

(16) Eby GA, Halcomb WW. Use of topical zinc to prevent recurrent herpes simplex infection: review of literature and suggested protocols. Med Hypotheses 1985;17:157–65.

(17) Prasad AS. Zinc: the biology and therapeutics of an ion. Ann Intern Med. 1996 Jul 15;125(2):142-4.

(18) National Institute of Health - Office of Dietary Supplements: http://ods.od.nih.gov/factsheets/cc/zinc.html#rda. Accessed December 19, 2007.

(19) Bryce-Smith D and Hodgkinson L: The Zinc Solution. Century Arrow, 1987.

(20) Bryce-Smith D: Zinc deficiency - the neglected factor. Chemistry in Britain, pp. 783-786, August, 1989.

(21) Bryce-Smith D: The Diagnosis of Zinc Deficiency. Felmore Ltd Health Publications No:118 - BNF.

(22) Bryce-Smith D and Simpson RID: Anorexia, depression and zinc deficiency. Lancet, ii:2162 1984.

(23) Simpson RID and Bryce-Smith D: Cutaneous manifestations of zinc deficiency during treatment by anticonvulsants. Br Med J, 290:1215-16, 1985.

(24) Schauss AG and Bryce-Smith D: Evidence of zinc deficiency in anorexia nervosa and bulimia nervosa. In: Nutrition and Brain Function, Ed: WB Essman, Karger, Basel, pp 151-162, 1987.

(25) Davies S: Zinc, nutrition and health. In: 1984-85 Yearbook of Nutritional Medicine Ed; J Bland, pp 113-152, Keats Publishing, New Canaan, Conn. 1985.

(26) Halstead JA, Smith JC: Plasma-zinc in health and disease. Lancet, i:322-24, 1970.

(27) Casper RC, Kirchner B, Sandstead HH, et al: An evaluation of trace metals, vitamins and minerals and taste function in anorexia nervosa. Am J Clin Nutr, 33:1801-08, 1980.

(28) http://www.uspharmacist.com/index.asp?show=article&page=8_1546.htm

(29) Chandra RK. Excessive intake of zinc impairs immune responses. *JAMA* 1984;252:1443.

(30) Jafek BW, Linschoten MR, Murrow BW. Anosmia after intranasal zinc gluconate use. *Am J Rhinol* 2004;18:137–41.

(31) Broun ER, Greist A, Tricot G, Hoffman R. Excessive zinc ingestion. A reversible cause of sideroblastic anemia and bone marrow depression. *JAMA* 1990;264:1441–3.

(32) Dawson EB, Albers J, McGanity WJ. Serum zinc changes due to iron supplementation in teen-age pregnancy. *Am J Clin Nutr* 1990;50:848–52.

118

(33) Crofton RW, Gvozdanovic D, Gvozdanovic S, et al. Inorganic zinc and the intestinal absorption of ferrous iron. *Am J Clin Nutr* 1989;50:141–4.

(34) Argiratos V, Samman S. The effect of calcium carbonate and calcium citrate on the absorption of zinc in healthy female subjects. *Eur J Clin Nutr* 1994;48:198–204.

(35) Spencer H, Norris C, Williams D. Inhibitory effects of zinc on magnesium balance and magnesium absorption in man. *J Am Coll Nutr* 1994;13:479–84.

(36) Brumas V, Hacht B, Filella M, Berthon G. Can N-acetyl-L-cysteine affect zinc metabolisms when used as a paracetamol antidote? *Agents Actions* 1992;36:278–88.

(40) Alaimo K, McDowell MA, Briefel RR, et al. Dietary intake of vitamins, minerals, and fiber of persons ages 2 months and over in the United States: Third National Health and Nutrition Examination Survey, Phase 1, 1988-91. Adv Data. 1994 Nov 14;(258):1-28.

Chapter 9 - Lactoferrin References

(1) Zhang GH, Mann DM, Tsai CM. Neutralization of endotoxin in vitro and in vivo by a human lactoferrin-derived peptide. Infect Immun 1999 Mar;67(3):1353-8.

(2) Lee WJ, Farmer JL, Hilty M, Kim YB. The Protective Effects of Lactoferrin Feeding against Endotoxin Lethal Shock in Germfree Piglets. Infect Immun Apr. 1999: Vol 66 No 4, 1421-1426.

(3) Zimecki M, Wlaszczyk A, Cheneau P, Brunel AS, Mazurier J, Spik G, Kubler A. Immunoregulatory effects of a nutritional preparation containing bovine lactoferrin taken orally by healthy individuals. Arch Immunol Ther Exp (Warsz) 1998;46(4):231-40.

(4) Yamauchi K, Wakabayashi H, Hashimoto S, Teraguchi S, Hayasawa H, Tomita M. Effects of orally administered bovine lactoferrin on the immune system of healthy volunteers. Adv Exp Med Biol 1998;443:261-5.

(5) Kruzel ML, Harari Y, Chen CY, Castro GA. The gut. A key metabolic organ protected by lactoferrin during experimental systemic inflammation in mice. Adv Exp Med Biol 1998;443:167-73.

(6) Defer MC, Dugas B, Picard O, Damais C. Impairment of circulating lactoferrin in HIV-1 infection. Cell Mol Biol (Noisy-le-grand) 1995 May;41(3):417-21.

(7) Puddu P, Borghi P, Gessani S, Valenti P, Belardelli F, Seganti (8) Antiviral effect of bovine lactoferrin saturated with metal ions on early steps of human immunodeficiency virus type 1 infection. Int J Biochem Cell Biol 1998 Sep;30(9):1055-62.

(9) Superti F, Ammendolia MG, Valenti P, Seganti L. Antirotaviral activity of milk proteins: lactoferrin prevents rotavirus infection in the enterocyte-like cell line HT-29. Med Microbiol Immunol (Berl) 1997 Oct;186(2-3):83-91.

(10) Harmsen MC, Swart PJ, de Bethune MP, Pauwels R, De Clercq E, The TH, Meijer DK. Antiviral effects of plasma and milk proteins: lactoferrin shows potent activity against both human immunodeficiency virus and human cytomegalovirus replication in vitro. J Infect Dis 1995 Aug;172(2):380-8.

(11) Swart PJ, Kuipers EM, Smit C, Van Der Strate BW, Harmsen MC, Meijer DK. lactoferrin. Antiviral activity of lactoferrin. Adv Exp Med Biol 1998;443:205-13.

(12) Dial EJ, Hall LR, Serna H, Romero JJ, Fox JG, Lichtenberger LM. Antibiotic properties of bovine lactoferrin on Helicobacter pylori. Dig Dis Sci 1998 Dec;43(12):2750-6.

(13) Bhimani RS, Vendrov Y, Furmanski P. Influence of lactoferrin feeding and injection against systemic staphylococcal infections in mice. J Appl Microbiol 1999 Jan;86(1):135-44.

(14) Percival M. Intestinal Health. Clin. Nutri. Insights. 1997, Vol 5. No 5, 1-6.

(15) Kuwata H, Yip TT, Tomita M, Hutchens TW. Direct evidence of the generation in human stomach of an antimicrobial peptide domain (lactoferricin) from ingested lactoferrin. Biochim Biophys Acta 1998 Dec 8;1429(1):129-41.

(16) Andersen JH, Jenssen H, Gutteberg TJ. Lactoferrin and lactoferricin inhibit Herpes simplex 1 and 2 infection and exhibit synergy when combined with acyclovir. Antiviral Res. 2003 May;58(3):209-15.

(17) Stella V, Postaire E. Evaluation of the antiradical protector effect of multifermented milk serum with reiterated dosage in rats. C R Seances Soc Biol Fil 1995;189(6):1191-7.

(18) Tsuda H, Sekine K, Nakamura J, Ushida Y, Kuhara T, Takasuka N, Kim DJ, Asamoto M, Baba-Toriyama H, Moore MA, Nishino H, Kakizoe T. Inhibition of azoxymethane initiated colon tumor and aberrant crypt foci development by bovine lactoferrin administration in F344 rats. Adv Exp Med Biol 1998;443:273-84.

(19) Ushida Y, Sekine K, Kuhara T, Takasuka N, Iigo M, Tsuda H. Inhibitory effects of bovine lactoferrin on intestinal polyposis in the Apc(Min) mouse. Cancer Lett 1998 Dec 25;134(2):141-5.

(20) Yoo YC, Watanabe S, Watanabe R, Hata K, Shimazaki K, Azuma I. Bovine lactoferrin and lactoferricin, a peptide derived from bovine lactoferrin, inhibit tumor metastasis in mice. Jpn J Cancer Res 1997 Feb;88(2):184-90.

(21) Sakamoto N. Antitumor effect of human lactoferrin against newly established human pancreatic cancer cell line SPA. Gan To Kagaku Ryoho 1998 Aug;25(10):1557-63.

120

Chapter 10 - Beta Glucan References

(1) Fitzpatrick FW, DiCarlo JF. Zymosan. In Annals of the New York Academy of Sciences, V.118., p.233-262.1964.

(2) Di Luzio NR: Immunopharmacolo~y of glucan : a broad spectrum enhancer of host defense mechanisms. Trends in Pharmacological Sciences 1983; 4: 344-347.

(3) Czop JK, Austen KF: A b-glucan inhibitable receptor on human monocytes: its identity with the phagocytic receptor for particulate activators of the alternative complement pathway. JImmunol 1985; 134: 2588-2593.

(4) Goldman R: Characteristics of the b-glucan receptor of murine macrophages. Exp Cel Res 1988; 174: 481-490.

(5) Janusz MJ, Austen KF, Czop JK. Isolation of a yeast heptaglucoside that inhibits monocyte phagocytosis of zymosan particles. The Journal of Immunology 198; 142.

(6) Hahn MG, Albersheim P: Host-pathogen interactions. XIV. Isolation and partial characterization of an elicitor from yeast extract. Plant Physiol 197X; 62: 107.

(7) Seljelid R, Figenschau Y, Bogwald J, et al. Evidence that tumor necrosis induced by aminated beta 1-3D polyglucose is mediated by a concerted action of local and systemic cytokines. Scand J Immunol. Dec1989;30(6):687-94.

(8) Bousquet M, Escoula L, Peuriere S, et al. Immunopharmacologic study in mice of 2 beta-1, 3, beta-1, 6 polysaccharides (scleroglucan and PSAT) on the activation of macrophages and T lymphocytes. Ann Rech Vet. 1989;20(2):165-73.

(9) Seljelid R, Figenschau Y, Bogwald J, et al. Evidence that tumor necrosis induced by aminated beta 1-3D polyglucose is mediated by a concerted action of local and systemic cytokines. Scand J Immunol. Dec1989;30(6):687-94.

(10) Kougias P, Wei D, Rice PJ, et al. Normal human fibroblasts express pattern recognition receptors for fungal (1-->3)-beta-D-glucans. Infect Immun. Jun2001;69(6):3933-8.

(11) Patchen M: Radioprotective effect of Oral Administration of NSC-24™. 1989. ImmuDyne, Inc. Unpublished.

(12) Patchen ML, D'Alesandro MM, Brook I, Blakely WF, McVittie TJ: Glucan: mechanisms involved in its "radioprotective" effect.. J Leuc Biol 1987; 42: 95-105.

(13) Bell S, Goldman VM, Bistrian BR, et al. Effect of beta-glucan from oats and yeast on serum lipids. Crit Rev Food Sci Nutr 1999;39:189-202

(14) Bell S, Goldman VM, Bistrian BR, et al. Effect of beta-glucan from oats and yeast on serum lipids. Crit Rev Food Sci Nutr 1999;39:189-202

(15) Behall KM, Scholfield DJ, Hallfrisch J. Effect of beta-glucan level in oat fiber extracts on blood lipids in men and women. J Am Coll Nutr 1997;16:46-51.

(16) Braaten JT, Wood PJ, Scott FW, et al. Oat beta-glucan reduces blood cholesterol concentration in hypercholesterolemic subjects. Eur J Clin Nutr 1994;48:465-74.

(17) Davidson MH, Dugan LD, Burns JH, et al. The hypocholesterolemic effects of beta-glucan in oatmeal and oat bran. A dose-controlled study. JAMA 1991;265:1833-9.

(18) Wood PJ. Physicochemical properties and physiological effects of the (1,3)(1,4)-beta-D-glucan from oats. Adv Exp Med Biol 1990;270:119-27.

(19) Uusitupa MI, Miettinen TA, Sarkkinen ES, et al. Lathosterol and other non-cholesterol sterols during treatment of hypercholesterolaemia with beta-glucan-rich oat bran. Eur J Clin Nutr 1997;51:607-11.

(20) Lia A, Hallmans G, Sandberg AS, et al. Oat beta-glucan increases bile acid excretion and a fiber-rich barley fraction increases cholesterol excretion in ileostomy subjects. Am J Clin Nutr 1995;62:1245-51.

(21) Bell S, Goldman VM, Bistrian BR, et al. Effect of beta-glucan from oats and yeast on serum lipids. Crit Rev Food Sci Nutr 1999;39:189-202

(22) Nicolosi R, Bell SJ, Bistrian BR, et al. Plasma lipid changes after supplementation with beta-glucan fiber from yeast. Am J Clin Nutr 1999;70:208-12.

(23) Behall KM, Scholfield DJ, Hallfrisch J. Effect of beta-glucan level in oat fiber extracts on blood lipids in men and women. J Am Coll Nutr 1997;16:46-51.

(24) Braaten JT, Wood PJ, Scott FW, et al. Oat beta-glucan reduces blood cholesterol concentration in hypercholesterolemic subjects. Eur J Clin Nutr 1994;48:465-74.

(25) Uusitupa MI, Ruuskanen E, Makinen E, et al. A controlled study on the effect of beta-glucan-rich oat bran on serum lipids in hypercholesterolemic subjects: relation to apolipoprotein E phenotype. J Am Coll Nutr 1992;11:651-9.

(26) Braaten JT, Scott FW, Wood PJ, et al. High beta-glucan oat bran and oat gum reduce postprandial blood glucose and insulin in subjects with and without type 2 diabetes. Diabet Med 1994;11:312-8.

(27) Wood PJ. Physicochemical properties and physiological effects of the (1,3)(1,4)-beta-D-glucan from oats. Adv Exp Med Biol 1990;270:119-27.

(28) Bourdon I, Yokoyama W, Davis P, et al. Postprandial lipid, glucose, insulin, and cholecystokinin responses in men fed barley pasta enriched with beta-glucan. Am J Clin Nutr 1999;69:55-63.

(29) Pick ME, Hawrysh ZJ, Gee MI. Oat bran concentrate bread products improve long-term control of diabetes: a pilot study. J Am Diet Assoc 1996;96:1254-61.

(30) Frey A, Giannasca KT, Weltzin R, et al. Role of the glycocalyx in regulating access of microparticles to apical plasma membranes of intestinal epithelial cells: implications for microbial attachment and oral vaccine targeting. J Exp Med. Sep1996;184(3):1045-59.

(31) Tsukagoshi S, Hashimoto Y, Fujii G, et al. Krestin (PSK). Cancer Treat Rev. Jun1984;11(2):131-55.

(32) Rylander R, Lin RH. (1-->3)-beta-D-glucan - relationship to indoor air-related symptoms, allergy and asthma. Toxicology. Nov 2000;152(1-3):47-52.

(33) Rylander R, et al. (1-->3)-beta-D-glucan may contribute to pollen sensitivity. Clin Exp Immunol. Mar 1999;115(3):383-4.

(34 The Acute Oral Toxicity Study of NSC-24 in Rats. Essex Testing Clinic. 1990, NJ, USA.

Chapter 11 - Thymic Protein A References

(1) Dean, Ward, MD and English, Jim, Thymic Protein A: Restoring Thymic Function for Immune Support, http://www.vrp.com/art/755.asp?c=1164308956843&k=/vrpsearch.asp&m=/includes/vrp.css&p=no&s=0

(2) Lau. C. Y. and Goldstein G. 1980. Functional effects of thymopoietin. J. Immunol. 124:1861.

(3) White, A. and Burton, P. 1979. Isolation from human plasma of a protein fraction with thymus hormone-like activity. Ann. N.Y. Acad. Sci. 332:1.

(4) Rosenbaum, M. E., Vojdani, A., Susser, M., Watson, C.M. Improved immune activation markers in chronic fatigue and immune dysfunction syndrome (CFIDS) patients treated with thymic protein A. Journal of Nutritional & Environmental Medicine 2001; 11: 241-7.

(5) South, James, "Thymus Gland, Its Overlooked But Vital Role," Vitamin Research News, November, 1999, Vol. 13:11, pp 1-5. 2. K. Kelly et al. "A pituitary-Thymus Connection During Aging." Ann. N.Y. Acad. Sci. 521, 88-98, 1988.

(6) Dean, Ward, MD. "The Neuroendocrine Theory of Aging Part IV—The Immune Homeostat." Vitamin Research News, October, 1999, Vol. 13:10, pp 1-11.

(7) Fabris, N., Mocchegiani, E., Muzzioli, M., and Provinciali, M. Neuroendocrine-thymus interactions: Perspectives for intervention in aging. In: Neuroimmunomodulation: Interventions in Aging and Cancer, Ann NY

Acad Sci, Vol 621, by Pierpaoli, W. and Spector, N.H., (eds). NY Acad Sci, New York, 1988, 72-87.

(8) Cardarelli, Nate. The role of a thymus-pineal axis in an immune mechanism of aging. J Theor Biol, 1990, 145: 397-405.

(9) Beardsley TR, Pierschbacher M, Wetzel GD, Hays EF. Induction of T-cell maturation by a cloned line of thymic epithelium (TEPI). Proc Natl Acad Sci USA 1983 Oct;80(19):6005-9.

(10) Hays EF, Beardsley TR. Immunologic effects of human thymic stromal grafts and cell lines. Clin Immunol Immunopathol 1984 Dec;33(3):381-90.

(11) Fabris, N., Mocchegiani, E., Muzzioli, M., and Provinciali, M. Role of zinc in neuroendocrine-immune interactions during aging. In: Physiological Senescence and Its Postponement, Ann New York Acad Sci, Vol 621, by Walter Pierpaoli and Nicola Fabris, (eds.),1991, NY Acad Sci, New York, 314-326.

(12) US Patent 5616554, http://www.freepatentsonline.com/5616554.html

Chapter 12 - Cimetidine References

(1) Devine SM, Wingard JR 1994, Viral infections in severely immunocompromised cancer patients. Support Care Cancer 1994 Nov;2(6):355-68.

(2) Van der Spuy S, Levy DW, Levin W 1980. Cimetidine in the treatment of herpes virus infections. S Afr Med J Jul 19;58(3):112-6.

(3) Kapinska-Mrowiecka M, Toruwski G: 1996. Efficacy of cimetidine in treatment of herpes zoster in the first 5 days from the moment of disease manifestation. Pol Tyg Lek Jun;51(23-26):338-9.

(4) Hayne ST, Mercer JB 1983. Herpes zoster:treatment with cemetidine. Can Med Assoc J Dec 15;129(12):1284-5.

(5) Komlos L, Notmann J, Arieli J, et.al. 1994. In vitro cell-mediated immune reactions in herpes zoster patients treated with cimetidine. Asian Pac J Allelrgy Immunol Jun;12(1):51-8.

(6) Miller A, Harel D, Laor A, Lahat N 1989. Cimetidine as an immunomodulator in the treatment of herpes zoster. J Neuroimmunol 1989 Mar;22(1):69-76.

(7) Kumar A, 1990. Cimetidine: an immunomodulator. DICP Mar;24(3):289-95.

(8) Kelly MD, King J, Cherian M, Dwerryhouse SJ, Finlay IG, Adams WJ, King DW, Lubowski D, Morris DL. 1999. Randomized Trial of Preoperative Cimetidine in Patients with Colorectal Carcinoma with Quantitative Assessment of Tumor-Associated Lymphocytes. Cancer Journal 85: 1658-63.

124

(9) Yilmaz, E, Alpsoy E, Basaran E. 1996. Cimetidine therapy for warts: a placebo-controlled, double-blind study. J Am Acad Dermatol Jun; 34(6):1005-7.

(10) Franco I 2000. Oral cemetidine for the management of genital and perigenital warts in children. J Urol Sep;164(3 Pt 2):1074-5.

(11) Adams WJ, Morris DL, Ross WB, Lubowski DZ, King DW, Peters L. , Cimetidine preserves non-specific immune function after colonic resection for cancer. Department of Surgery, St George Hospital, Kogarah, New South Wales, Australia. Aust N Z J Surg 1994 Dec;64(12):847-52

(12) Adams WJ, Lawson JA, Nicholson SE, Cook TA, Morris DL. ,The growth of carcinogen-induced colon cancer in rats is inhibited by cimetidine., Department of Surgery, St George Hospital, University of New South Wales, Sydney, Australia. Eur J Surg Oncol 1993 Aug;19(4):332-5

(13) Matsumoto S, Imaeda Y, Umemoto S, Kobayashi K, Suzuki H, Okamoto T., Cimetidine increases survival of colorectal cancer patients with high levels of sialyl, Lewis-X and sialyl Lewis-A epitope expression on tumour cells Department of Surgery, Second Teaching Hospital, School of Medicine, Fujita Health University, 3-6-10 Otohbashi, Nakagawa-ku, Nagoya 454-8509, Japan. Br J Cancer 2002 Jan 21;86(2):161-7

(14) Effect of cimetidine on survival after gastric cancer. Tonnesen H, Knigge U, Bulow S, Damm P, Fischerman K, Hesselfeldt P, Hjortrup A, Pedersen IK, Pedersen VM, Siemssen OJ, et al. Hvidovre Hospital, Copenhagen, Denmark. Lancet 1988 Oct 29;2(8618):990-2

(15) Tagemet To Treat Herpes And Shingles, Life Extension Magazine March 2001

(15) Avella J, Binder H, Madsen J, Ashkenase P. Effect of histamine H2 receptor antagonists on delayed hypersensitivity. Lancet 1978:1:624-626.

(16) Dohil M, Prendiville JS. Treatment of Molluscum contagiosum with oral cimetidine: clinical experience on 13 patients. Pediatric Dermatol 13:310-312.

(17) Br J Cancer 2002 Jan 21;86(2):161-7

(18) Eur J Cancer Clin Oncol 1988 Feb;24(2):161-7

(19) Lancet 1988 Oct 29;2(8618):990-2

(20) Am J Surg 1986 Feb;151(2):249-55

(21) Aust N Z J Surg 1994 Dec;64(12):847-52

(22) Eur J Surg Oncol 1993 Aug;19(4):332-5

(23) Drug Intell Clin Pharm 1987 Oct;21(10):803-5

(24) Clin Immunol Immunopathol 1988 Jul;48(1):50-60

125

(25) Can Med Assoc J 1983 Dec 15;129(12):1284-5

(26) Support Care Cancer 1994 Nov;2(6):355-68

(27) S Afr Med J 1980 Jul 19;58(3):112-6

(28) J Am Acad Dermatol 1996 Jun;34(6):1005-7

(29) DICP 1990 Mar;24(3):289-95

(30) J Neuroimmunol 1989 Mar;22(1):69-76

(31) Asian Pac J Allergy Immunol 1994 Jun;12(1):51-8

(32) J Urol 2000 Sep;164(3 Pt 2):1074-5

(33) Pol Tyg Lek 1996 Jun;51(23-26):338-9

(34) Cancer 1999 Apr 15;85(8):1658-63

(35) Tonnesen H, Knigge U, Bulow S, Damm P, Fischerman K, Hesselfeldt P, Hjortrup A, Pedersen IK, Pedersen VM, Siemssen OJ. Effect of cimetadine on survival after gastric cancer. Lancet 1988 Oct 29;2(8618):990-2.

(36) Adams WJ, Morris DL. Short-course cimetadine and survival with colorectal cancer. Lancet. 1994 Dec 24-31;344(8939-8940):1768-9.

(37) Matsumoto S, Imaeda Y, Umemoto S, Kobayashi K, Suzuki H, Okamoto T. Cimetadine increases survival of colorectal cancer patients with high levels of sialyl Lewis-X and sialyl Lewis-A epitope expression on tumour cells. Brit J Can 2002 (86) 161-167.

(38) Kobayashi K, Matsumoto S, Morishima T, Kawabe T, Okamoto T. Cimetadine inhibits cancer cell adhesion to endothelial cells and prevents metastasis by blocking E-selectin expression. Cancer Res. 2000 Jul 15;60(14):3978-84.

(39) Adams WJ, Lawson JA, Morris DL. Cimetadine inhibits in vivo growth of human colon cancer and reverses histamine stimulated in vitro and in vivo growth. Gut 1994 Nov;35(11):1632-6.

(40) Siegers CP, Hiltl DM, Stich R. Cimetadine hemmt das Tumorzellwachstum. Therapie-woche. 1995 (36) 2110-2114.

(41) Melmon KL, Bourne HR, Weinstein Y, Sela MD. Receptors for histamine can be detected on the surface of selected leukocytes. Science 1972 (177) 707.

(42) Rocklin RE, Greineder DK, Melmon KL. Histamine induced suppressor factor (HSF) Further studies on the nature of the stimulus and the cell which produces it. Cell Immunol 1979 (44) 404-415.

(43) Hansbrough J, Zapata-Sirvent R, Bender E. Prevention of alterations in postoperative lymphocyte subpopulations by cimetadine and ibuprofen. Am. J surg 1986 151, 249-255.

(44) Adams W. Cimetadine preserves immune function after colonic resection of cancer. Aust. NZ J. Surg 1994 64, 847-852.

(45) Adams WJ, Lawson JA, Nicholson SE, Cook TA, Morris DL. The growth of carcinogen-induced colon cancer in rats is inhibited by cimetadine. Eur J Surg Oncol 1993 Aug;19 (4):332-5.

(46) Harrison JC, Dean PJ, El-Zeky F, Vander Zwaag R. From Dukes through Jass: Pathological prognostic indicators in rectal cancer. Hum. Path. 1994 (25) 495-498.

(47) Morris DL, Adams WJ. Cimetadine and colorectal cancer-old drug, new use? Nat Med. 1995 Dec;1(12):1243-4.

(48) Uchida A. Biological significance of autologous tumour killing activity and its induction therapy. Cancer Immun. Immunother 1993 (37) 75-83.

(49) American Cancer Society website - Statistics section. Cimetadine (Tagamet®) For Cancer Treatment, LE Magazine July 2002

(50) Bense L, Marcusson JA, Ramsten T, Effect of Cimetidine on herpes zoster infection, Drug Intell Clin Pharm, 1987 Oct. 21 (10):803-5

(51) Armitage, JO and Sidner, RD. Antitumour effect of cimetidine? The Lancet, pages 882-883, April 21, 1979

(52) Brockmeyer, NH and others. Immunomodulatory properties of cimetidine in ARC patients. Clinical Immunology and Immunopathology, number 48, pages 50-60, 1988

(53) Tonnesen, H and others. Effect of cimetidine on survival after gastric cancer. The Lancet, October 29, pages 990-991, 1988.

(54)Gifford, RRM and Tilberg, AF. Histamine type-2 antagonist immune modulation II. Cimetidine and ranitidine increase interleukin-2 production. Surgery, volume 102, number 2, pages 242-247, August, 1987.

(55) Allen, JI and others. Cimetidine modulates natural killer cell function of patients with chronic lymphocytic leukemia. Journal of Laboratory Clinical Medicine, volume 109, number 4, pages 396-401, April 1987.

(56) White, WB and Ballow, M. Modulation of suppressor-cell activity by cimetidine in patients with common variable hypogammaglobu- linemia. The New England Journal of Medicine, volume 312, number 4, pages 198-202, January 24, 1985.

(57) http://www.nlm.nih.gov/medlineplus/druginfo/medmaster/a682256.html

Chapter 13 - Coconut Oil References

(1) Ascherio A., Munger K.L., Lenette E.T., Spiegelman D., Hernan M.A., Olek M.J., Hankinson S.E., and Hunter, D.J. Epstein-Barr virus antibodies and risk of multiple sclerosis: a prospective study. JAMA 286(24:3127-9, Dec. 26th, 2001.

(2) Awad AB. Effect of dietary lipids on composition and glucose utilization by rat adipose tissue. Journal of Nutrition 111:34-39, 1981.

(3) Bierenbaum JL, Green DP, Florin A, Fleishman AI, Caldwell AB. Modified-fat dietary management of the young male with coronary disease: a five-year report. Journal of the American Medical Association 202:1119-1123;1967.

(4) Beuchat LA. Comparison of antiviral activities of potassium sorbate, sodium benzoate and glycerol and sucrose esters of fatty acids. Appi. Environ. Microbiol. 39:1178, 1980.

(5) Blackburn GL, Kater G, Mascioli EA, Kowalchuk M, Babayan VK, kBistrian BR. A reevaluation of coconut oil's effect on serum cholesterol and atherogenesis. The Journal of the Philippine Medical Association 65:144-152;1989.

(6) Boddie RL and Nickerson SE. Evaluation of postmilking teat germicides containing Lauricidin, saturated fatty acids, and lactic acid. J. Dairy Sci. 75(6):1725-30, 1992.

(7) Cohen SS. Strategy for the chemotherapy of infectious diseases. Science 197:431, 1977

(8) Dayrit, Conrado S. MD., Coconut Oil in Health and Disease: Its and Monolaurin's Potential as Cure for HIV / AIDS, XXXVII Cocotech Meeting, Chennai, India, July 25, 2000

(9) Dulbecco A. Interference with viral multi- plication. In: Virology, Dulbecco, A. and Ginsberg, H. edit, Harper & Row, Philadelphia, 1980.

(10) Enig, M. Coconut: In support of good health in the 21st century. 1999. www.mercola.com/2001/jul/28/ coconut_health.htm.

(11) Enig, MG: Coconut Oil: An Anti-bacterial, Anti-viral Ingredient for Food, Nutrition and Health., AVOC Lauric Symposium, Manila, Philippines, Oct. 17, 1997.

(12) Eraly MG. IV. Coconut oil and heart attack. Coconut and Coconut Oil in Human Nutrition, Proceedings. Symposium on Coconut and Coconut Oil in Human Nutrition. 27 March 1994. Coconut Development Board, Kochi, India, 1995, pp 63-64.

(13) Fife, B. The Healing Miracles of Coconut Oil. Colorado Springs: Health Wise Pub; 2003:15.

(14) Fletcher RD, Albers AC, Albertson JN, Kabara JJ. Effects of monoglycerides on mycoplasma pneumoniae growth, in The Pharmacological

Effect of Lipids II (JJ Kabara, ed) American Oil Chemists' Society, Champaign IL, 1985, pp.59-63.

(15) Han, J. et al. Medium-chain oil reduces fat mass and down-regulates expression of adipogenic genes in rats. Obes Res 2003, 11:734-44.

(16) Hierholzer, J.C. and Kabara, J.J. In vitro effects of monolaurin compounds on enveloped RNA and DNA viruses. Journal of Food Safety 4:1-12;1982.

(17) Hierholzer, JC and Kabara, JJ: In vitro effects of monolaurin compounds on enveloped RNA and DNA viruses., J. Food Safety 4:1-12, 1982

(18) Isaacs CE, Thormar H. Membrane-disruptive effect of human milk: inactivation of enveloped viruses. Journal of Infectious Diseases 154:966-971;1986.

(19) Isaacs CE, Thormar H. The role of milk-derived antimicrobial lipids as antiviral and antibacterial agents in Immunology of Milk and the Neonate (Mestecky J, et al, eds) Plenum Press, New York, 1991.

(20) Isaacs CE. The antimicrobial function of milk lipids. Adv. Nutr. Res. 10:271-85, 2001.

(21) Isaacs CE, Schneidman K. Enveloped Viruses in Human and Bovine Milk are Inactivated by Added Fatty Acids(FAs) and Monoglycerides(MGs). FASEB Journal. Abstract 5325, p.A1288, 1991.

(22) Isaacs CE, Kashyap S, Heird WC, Thormar H. Antiviral and antibacterial lipids in human milk and infant formula feeds. Archives of Disease in Childhood 65:861-864;1990.

(23) Isaacs CE, Litov RE, Marie P, Thormar H. Addition of lipases to infant formulas produces antiviral and antibacterial activity. Journal of Nutritional Biochemistry 3:304-308;1992.

(24) Ismail-Cassim, N et al. Inhibition of the uncoating of bovine enterovirus by short chain fatty acids. J. Gen. Virol. 71(10):2283-9, 1990.

(25) Kabara JJ. Fatty acids and derivatives as antimicrobial agents -- A review, in The Pharmacological Effect of Lipids (JJ Kabara, ed) American Oil Chemists' Society, Champaign IL, 1978.

(26) Kabara JJ et al. Fatty acids and derivatives as antimicrobial agents. Antimicrob. Agents Chemother. 2:23, 1972

(27) Kabara JJ. Inhibition of staphylococcus aureaus in The Pharmacological Effect of Lipids II (JJ Kabara, ed) American Oil Chemists' Society, Champaign IL, 1985, pp.71-75.

(28) Kabara JJ. Lipids as host-resistance factors of human milk. Nutr. Rev. 38:65, 1980.

(29) Kabara, J. Health oils from the tree of life (Nutritional and health aspects of coconut oil). www.coconutoil.com/research.htm.

(30) Kasai, M. Comparison of diet-induced thermogenesis of foods containing medium- versus long-chain triacylglycerols. J Nutr Sci Vitaminol (Tokyo) 2002, 48:536-40.

(31) Kaunitz H, Dayrit CS. Coconut oil consumption and coronary heart disease. Philippine Journal of Internal Medicine 30:165-171;1992.

(32) Keys A, Anderson JT, Grande F. Prediction of serum-cholesterol responses of man to changes in the diet. Lancet, 959;1957.

(33) Kohn A. et al. Unsaturated free fatty acids inactivated animal envelope viruses. Arch. Virol. 66:301-306, 1980

(34) Kurup PA, Rajmohan T. II. Consumption of coconut oil and coconut kernel and the incidence of atherosclerosis. Coconut and Coconut Oil in Human Nutrition, Proceedings. Symposium on Coconut and Coconut Oil in Human Nutrition. 27 March 1994. Coconut Development Board, Kochi, India, 1995, pp 35-59.

(35) Kumar, P. The role of coconut and coconut oil in coronary heart disease in Kerala, South India. Trop Doct 1997, 27:215-17. 7. 2 op. cit., 58.

(36) Lim-Sylianco CY. Anticarcinogenic effect of coconut oil. The Philippine Journal of Coconut Studies 12:89-102;1987.

(37) Mendis S, Wissler RW, Bridenstine RT, Podbielski FJ. The effects of replacing coconut oil with corn oil on human serum lipid profiles and platelet derived factors active in atherogenesis. Nutrition Reports International 40:No.4;Oct.1989.

(38) Mendis, S. and Kumarasunderam, R. The effect of daily consumption of coconut fat and soya-bean fat on plasma lipids and lipoproteins of young normolipidaemic men. Br J Nutr 1990, 63:547-52.

(39) Prior IA, Davidson F, Salmond CE, Czochanska Z. Cholesterol, coconuts, and diet on Polynesian atolls: a natural experiment: the Pukapuka and Tokelau Island studies. American Journal of Clinical Nutrition 34:1552-1561;1981.

(40) Projan SJ, Brown-Skrobot S, Schlievert PM, Vandenesch F, Novick RP. Glycerol monolaurate inhibits the production of beta-lactamase, toxic shock toxin-1, and other staphylococcal exoproteins by interefering with signal transduction. Journal of Bacteriology. 176:4204-4209;1994.

(41) Rabia S. et al. Inactivation of vesicular stomatitis virus by photosensitization following incubation with a pyrene-fatty acid. Febs. Let. 270(12):9-10, 1990.

(42) Sands JA et al. Antiviral effects of fatty acids and derivatives. In: Pharmacological Effects of Lipids. Am. Oil Chem. Soc: Champaign, 1979;75.

130

(43) Sands J et al. Extreme sensitivity of enveloped viruses, including herpes simplex, to long chain unsaturated monoglycerides and alcohols. Antimicrobial Agents and Chemotherapy 15(1):67-73, 1979.

(44) Sircar, S. and Kansra, U. Choice of cooking oils-myths and realities. J Indian Med Assoc 1998, 96:304-07.

(45) Silver RK et al. Factors in human milk interfering with influenza-virus activities. Science 123:932-933, 1956

(46) Simmons A. Herpes virus and multiple sclerosis. Herpes 8(3):60-3, Nov. 2001

(47) Smith RL. The Cholesterol Conspiracy. Warren H Green Inc. St. Louis, Missouri, 1991.

(48) St-Onge, M. et al. Medium-chain triglycerides increase energy expenditure and decrease adiposity in overweight men. Obes Res 2003, 11:395-402.

(49) St-Onge, M. and Jones, P. Physiological effects of medium-chain triglycerides: potential agents in the prevention of obesity. J Nutr 2002, 132:329-32.

(50) Tayag E, Dayrit CS, Santiago EG, Manalo MA, Alban PN, Agdamag DM, Adel AS, Lazo S and Espallardo N: Monolaurin and Coconut Oil as Monotherapy for HIV-AIDS, Pilot Trial. For Publication.

(51) Thormar H, Isaacs EC, Brown HR, Barshatzky MR, Pessolano T. Inactivation of enveloped viruses and killing of cells by fatty acids and monoglycerides. Antimicrobial agents and chemotherapy 1987;31:27-31.

(52) Welsh JK, May JT. Anti-infective properties of breast milk. J. Pediatrics 94, 1-9, 1979.

Chapter 14 - BHT References

(1) Snipes W, Person S, Keith A, Cupp J. Butylated hydroxytoluene inactivates lipid-containing viruses. *Science*. 1975;188(4183):64-6.

(2) Brugh M Jr. Butylated hydroxytoluene protects chickens exposed to Newcastle disease virus. *Science*. 1977;197(4310):1291-2.

(3) Kim KS, Moon HM, Sapienza V, Carp RI, Pullarkat R. Inactivation of cytomegalovirus and Semliki Forest virus by butylated hydroxytoluene. *J Infect Dis* 1978;138(1):91-4.

(4) Pirtle EC, Sacks JM, Nachman RJ. Antiviral effectiveness of butylated hydroxytoluene against pseudorabies (Aujeszky's disease) virus in cell culture, mice, and swine. *Am J Vet Res*. 1986;47(9):1892-5.

(5) Richards JT, Katz ME, Kern ER. Topical butylated hydroxytoluene treatment of genital herpes simplex virus infections of guinea pigs. *Antiviral Res* 1985;5(5):281-90.

(6) Aloia RC, Jensen FC, Curtain CC, Mobley PW, Gordon LM. Lipid composition and fluidity of the human immunodeficiency virus. *Proc Natl Acad Sci U S A* 1988;85(3):900-4.

(7) Chetverikova LK, Ki'ldivatov II, Inozemtseva LI, Kramskaia TA, Filippov VK, Frolov BA. Factors of antiviral resistance in the pathogenesis of influenza in mice [in Russian]. *Vestn Akad Med Nauk SSSR* 1989;(11):63-8.

(8) Pearson D, Shaw S. *Life Extension: A Practical Scientific Approach*. New York, NY: Warner Books, Inc.; 1982:206-207.

(9) Mann JA, Fowkes SW. *Wipe Out Herpes with BHT*. Manhattan Beach, Calif: MegaHealth Society; 1983.
(10) Lanigan RS, Yamarik TA, Final report on the safety assessment of BHT, Int. J. Toxicol., 2002:21 Suppl 2:19-94

(11) Shlian DM, Goldstone J, Toxicity of butylated hydroxytoluene, N Engl J Med, 1986; 34; 648-649

(12)
http://www.vrp.com/showdoc.asp?c=1161225336828&k=/vrpsearch.asp&m=
/includes/vrp.css&p=no&s=0

Chapter 15 - Lysine References

(1) Thien DJ, Hurt WC, "Lysine as a prophylactic agent in the treatment of recurrent herpes simplex labialis" Oral Surg Oral Med Oral Pathol., 1984 Dec; 58(6) 659-66

(2) Milman N, Scheibel J, Jessen O, "Lysine prophylaxis in recurrent herpes simplex labialis: a double-blind, controlled crossover study." Acta Derm Venereol., 1980; 60(1): 85-7

(3) Griffith RS, Walsh DE, Myrmel KH, Thompson RW, Behforooz A, "Success of L-lysine therapy in frequently recurrent herpes simplex infection. Treatment and proophylaxis.," Dermatologica., 1978; 175(4): 183-90

(4) Griffin RS, Norins AL, Kagan C, "A Multicentered study of lysine therapy in Herpes simplex infection", Dermatologica, 1978; 156(5):257-67

(5) DiGiovanna JJ, Blank H, "Failure of lysine in frequently recurrent herpes simplex infection". Treatment and prophylaxis, Arch. Dermatol., 1984 Jan;120(1):48-51

(6) Kagan, C. "Lysine Therapy for Herpes Simplex", The Lancet, 1:137 26 Jan 1974

(7) Olshevsky, V., Becher V. Virology 1970, 40, 948

132

(8) Kaplan, A.S., Shimano, H., Ben-Porat, T. ibid p. 90.

(9) Agricultural Handbook, 1-23, U.S. Department of Agriculture

(10) McCune MA, Perry HO, Muller SA, O'Fallon WM. (2005). "Treatment of recurrent herpes simplex infections with L-lysine monohydrochloride". *Cutis.* 34 (4): 366-373.

(11) Griffith RS, Walsh DE, Myrmel KH, Thompson RW, Behforooz A. (1987). "Success of L-lysine therapy in frequently recurrent herpes simplex infection. Treatment and prophylaxis". *Dermatologica.* 175 (4): 183-190.

(12) Griffith RS, Norins AL, Kagan C. (1978). "A multicentered study of lysine therapy in Herpes simplex infection". *Dermatologica.* 156 (5): 257-267.

(13) Flodin NW. The metabolic roles, pharmacology, and toxicology of lysine. *J Am Coll Nutr* 1997;16:7–21 [review].

Chapter 16 - Garlic References

(1) Riddle JM. Garlic's history as a medicine. Paper presented at: American Herbal Products Association International Carlic Symposium; July 31, 2001.

(2) Heber D. Vegetables, fruits and phyto-estrogens in the prevention of diseases. J Postgrad Med. 2004 Apr;50(2):145-9.

(3) Atmaca G. Antioxidant effects of sulfur-containing amino acids. Yonsei Med J. 2004 Oct 31;45(5):776-88.

(4) Kempaiah RK, Srinivasan K. Influence of dietary curcumin, capsaicin and garlic on the antioxidant status of red blood cells and the liver in high-fat-fed rats. Ann Nutr Metab. 2004 September ;48(5):314-20.

(5) Kempaiah RK, Srinivasan K. Antioxidant status of red blood cells and liver in hypercholesterolemic rats fed hypolipidemic spices. Int J Vitam Nutr Res. 2004 May;74(3):199-208.

(6) Perez-Severiano F, Rodriguez-Perez M, Pedraza-Chaverri J, et al. S-Allylcysteine, a garlic-derived antioxidant, ameliorates quinolinic acid-induced neurotoxicity and oxidative damage in rats. Neurochem Int. 2004 Dec;45(8):1175-83.

(7) Maldonado PD, Barrera D, Rivero I, et al. Antioxidant S-allylcysteine prevents gentamicin-induced oxidative stress and renal damage. Free Radic Biol Med. 2003 Aug 1;35(3):317-24.

(8) Sovova M, Sova P. Pharmaceutical importance of Allium sativum L. 5. Hypolipemic effects in vitro and in vivo. Ceska Slov Farm. 2004 May;53(3):117-23.

(9) Durak A, Ozturk HS, Olcay E, Guven C. Effects of garlic extract supplementation on blood lipid and antioxidant parameters and atherosclerotic plaque formation process in cholesterol-fed rabbits. J Herb Pharmcother. 2002;2(2):19-32.

(10) Budoff MJ, Takasu J, Flores FR, et al. Inhibiting progression of coronary calcification using aged garlic extract in patients receiving statin therapy: a preliminary study. Prev Med. 2004 Nov;39(5):985-91.

(11) Wilburn AJ, King DS, Glisson J, Rockhold RW, Wofford MR. The natural treatment of hypertension. J Clin Hypertens.(Greenwich.) 2004 May;6(5):242-8.

(12) Durak I, Kavutcu M, Aytac B, et al. Effects of garlic extract consumption on blood lipid and oxidant/antioxidant parameters in humans with high blood cholesterol. J Nutr Biochem. 2004 Jun;15(6):373-7.

(13) Sengupta A, Ghosh S, Bhattacharjee S. Allium vegetables in cancer prevention: an overview. Asian Pac J Cancer Prev. 2004 Jul;5(3):237-45.

(14) Hassan HT. Ajoene (natural garlic compound): a new anti-leukaemia agent for AML therapy. Leuk Res. 2004 Jul;28(7):667-71.

(15) Ledezma E, Apitz-Castro R, Cardier J. Apoptotic and anti-adhesion effect of ajoene, a garlic derived compound, on the murine melanoma B16F10 cells: possible role of caspase-3 and the alpha(4)beta(1) integrin. Cancer Lett. 2004 Mar 31;206(1):35-41.

(16) Tilli CM, Stavast-Kooy AJ, Vuerstaek JD, et al. The garlic-derived organosulfur component ajoene decreases basal cell carcinoma tumor size by inducing apoptosis. Arch Dermatol Res. 2003 Jul;295(3):117-23.

(17) Xu B, Monsarrat B, Gairin JE, Girbal-Neuhauser E. Effect of ajoene, a natural antitumor small molecule, on human 20S proteasome activity in vitro and in human leukemic HL60 cells. Fundam Clin Pharmacol. 2004 Apr;18(2):171-80.

(18) Lu HF, Sue CC, Yu CS, et al. Diallyl disulfide (DADS) induced apoptosis undergo caspase-3 activity in human bladder cancer T24 cells. Food Chem Toxicol. 2004 Oct;42(10):1543-52.

(19) Wu CC, Chung JG, Tsai SJ, Yang JH, Sheen LY. Differential effects of allyl sulfides from garlic essential oil on cell cycle regulation in human liver tumor cells. Food Chem Toxicol. 2004 Dec;42(12):1937-47.

(20) Sengupta A, Ghosh S, Bhattacharjee S, Das S. Indian food ingredients and cancer prevention - an experimental evaluation of anticarcinogenic effects of garlic in rat colon. Asian Pac J Cancer Prev. 2004 Apr;5(2):126-32.

(21) Zlotogorski HA, Littner M. Potential risks, adverse effects and drug interactions associated with herbal medicine in dental patients. Refuat Hapeh Vehashinayim. 2004 Apr;21(2):25-41, 97.

(22) Ciocon JO, Ciocon DG, Galindo DJ. Dietary supplements in primary care. Botanicals can affect surgical outcomes and follow-up. Geriatrics. 2004 Sep;59(9):20-4.

134

(23) Hsing AW, Chokkalingam AP, Gao YT, Madigan MP, Deng J, Gridley G, Fraumeni JF Jr. Allium vegetables and risk of prostate cancer: a population-based study. J Natl Cancer Inst. 2002 Nov 6;94(21):1648-51

(24) Durak I, Aytac B, Atmaca Y, Devrim E, Avci A, Erol C, Oral D. Effects of garlic extract consumption on plasma and erythrocyte antioxidant parameters in atherosclerotic patients. Life Sci. 2004 Sep 3;75(16):1959-66.

(25) Saravanan G, Prakash J. Effect of garlic (Allium sativum) on lipid peroxidation in experimental myocardial infarction in rats. J Ethnopharmacol. 2004 Sep;94(1):155-8.

(26) Weber ND, Andersen DO, et al. In vitro virucidal effects of Allium sativum (garlic) extract and compounds. *Planta Med.* 1992 Oct;58(5):417-23.

(27) Guo NL, Lu DP, et al. Demonstration of the anti-viral activity of garlic extract against human cytomegalovirus in vitro. *Chin Med J (Engl).* 1993 Feb;106(2):93–6.

(28) Josling P. Preventing the common cold with a garlic supplement: A double-blind, placebo-controlled survey. *Adv Ther* . 2001 Jul;18(4):189–93.

(29) Kyo E, Uda N, et al. Immunomodulatory effects of aged garlic extract. *J Nutr* . 2001 Mar;131(3s):1075S – 9S.

(30) Koch HP, Lawson LD (eds). *Garlic: The Science and Therapeutic Application of Allium sativaum L and Related Species,* 2d ed. Baltimore: Williams and Wilkins, 1996, 62–4.

(31) Warshafsky S, Kamer R, Sivak S. Effect of garlic on total serum cholesterol: A meta-analysis. *Ann Int Med* 1993;119:599–605.

(32) Silagy C, Neil A. Garlic as a lipid-lowering agent—a meta-analysis. *J R Coll Phys* London 1994;28:39–45.

(33) Neil HA, Silagy CA, Lancaster T, et al. Garlic powder in the treatment of moderate hyperlipidaemia: A controlled trial and a meta-analysis. *J R Coll Phys* 1996;30:329–34.

(24) McCrindle BW, Helden E, Conner WT. Garlic extract therapy in children with hypercholesterolemia. *Arch Pediatr Adolesc Med* 1998;152:1089–94.

(35) Isaacsohn JL, Moser M, Stein EA, et al. Garlic powder and plasma lipids and lipoproteins. *Arch Intern Med* 1998;158:1189–94.

(36) Berthold HK, Sudhop T, von Bergmann K. Effect of a garlic oil preparation on serum lipoproteins and cholesterol metabolism. *JAMA* 1998;279:1900–2.

(37) Legnani C, Frascaro M, Guazzaloca G, et al. Effects of a dried garlic preparation on fibrinolysis and platelet aggregation in healthy subjects. *Arzneim-Forsch Drug Res* 1993;43:119–22.

(38) Silagy CA, Neil HA. A meta-analysis of the effect of garlic on blood pressure. *J Hyperten* 1994;12:463–8.

(39) Kleijnen J, Knipschild P, Ter Riet G. Garlic, onion and cardiovascular risk factors: A review of the evidence from human experiments with emphasis on commercially available preparations. *Br J Clin Pharmacol* 1989;28:535–44.

(40) Koscielny J, Klüendorf D, Latza R, et al. The antiatherosclerotic effect of *Allium sativum. Atherosclerosis* 1999;144:237–49.

(41) Hughes BG, Lawson LD. Antimicrobial effects of *Allium sativum* L. (garlic), *Allium ampeloprasum* L. (elephant garlic) and *Allium cepa* L. (onion), garlic compounds and commercial garlic supplement products. *Phytother Res* 1991;5:154–8.

(42) Dorant E, van den Brandt PA, Goldbohm RA, et al. Garlic and its significance for the prevention of cancer in humans: A critical review. *Br J Cancer* 1993;67:424–9.

(43) Fleishauer AT, Poole C, Arab L. Garlic consumption and cancer prevention: meta-analyses of colorectal and stomach cancers. *Am J Clin Nutr* 2000;72:1047–52.

(44) Brown DJ. *Herbal Prescriptions for Better Health.* Rocklin, CA: Prima Publishing, 1996, 97–109.

(45) Blumenthal M, Busse WR, Goldberg A, et al. (eds). *The Complete Commission E Monographs: Therapeutic Guide to Herbal Medicines.* Boston, MA: Integrative Medicine Communications, 1998, 134.

(46) Burnham BE: Garlic as a possible risk for postoperative bleeding. Plast Reconst Surg 1995; 95:213.

(47) Rose KD, Croissant PD, Parliament CF et al: Spontaneous spinal epidural hematoma with associated platelet dysfunction from excessive garlic ingestion: a case report. Neurosurg 1990; 26:880-882.

(48) Sunter W: Warfarin and garlic. Pharm J 1991; 246:722.

(49) Piscitelli SC, Burstein, Welden et al: Garlic supplements decrease saquinavir plasma concentrations [abstract]. 8th Conference on Retroviruses and Opportunistic Infections, Feb 4-8, 2001, Chicago, Illinois. Abstract 743.

(50) Gurley BJ, Gardner SF, Hubbard MA et al: Cytochrome P450 phenotypic ratios for predicting herb-drug interactions in humans. Clin Pharmacol Ther 2002; 72(3):276-287.

(51) Apitz-Castro R, Escalante J, Vargas R et al: Ajoene, the antiplatelet principle of garlic, synergistically potentiates the antiaggregatory action of prostacyclin, forskolin, indomethacin, and dypiridamole on human platelets. Thromb Res 1986; 42:303-311.

(52) Tsuei; Julia J., US Patent 4,795,636, Issued on January 3, 1989

136

(53) Bulatov, et al., 28 Sovietskaia Meditsina 86 (Dec. 1965) (Russian version with English summary enclosed).

(54) Esanu, "Recent Advances in the Chemotherapy of Herpes Virus Infections," 32 Virologie 57 (Jan.-Mar. 1981).

(55) Sekeley, et al., "Anti-Viral Activity of Azathymidine and Uracil Methyl Sulphone", 211 Nature 1260 (1966).

(56) Tsai, et al., "Antiviral Properties of Garlic: In Vitro Effects on Influenza B, Herpes Simplex and Coxsackie Viruses", 1985 Planta Medica No. 5,357 (Oct. 1985).

(57) Tsuei, J. Method for treating genital and oral herpes. International Publication Number WO97/03203. International Patent Classification: A61K 35/78, June 4, 1987.

(58) Abdullah, T., Kirkpatrick, D., D. et al. Enhancement of Natural *Onkologie* 21:52-53, 1989.

(59) Lau BH; Yamasaki T; Gridley DS, Garlic compounds modulate macrophage and T-lymphocyte functions, Mol Biother, 1991 Jun, 3:2, 103-7

(60) Ackermann RT, Mulrow CD, Ramirez G, Gardner CD, Morbidoni L, Lawrence VA. Garlic shows promise for improving some cardiovascular risk factors. Arch Intern Med 2001;161:813-24.

(61) Blumenthal M, Goldberg A, Brinckmann J (eds). *Herbal Medicine: Expanded Commission E Monographs.* 1st ed., (Newton, MA: Integrative Medicine Communications. 2000).

(62) Tyler, Varro., Brady, Lynn., Robbers, James., *Pharmacognosy.* 9th ed., (Philadelphia, Lea & Febiger, 1988

(63) World Health Organization. *WHO Monographs on Selected Medicinal Plants*, Vol. 1. (Geneva, Switzerland: World Health Organization. 1999).

(64) Blumenthal M, Busse W, Goldberg A, Gruenwald J, Hall T, Riggins CW, Rister RS (eds.). *The Complete German Commission E Monographs: Therapeutic Guide to Herbal Medicines.* S. Klein, R.S. Rister (trans.). 1st ed., (Austin, TX: American Botanical Council. 1998).

(65) European Scientific Cooperative on Phytotherapy. *ESCOP Monographs on the Medicinal Uses of Plant Drugs.* 1st ed., (Exeter, U.K.: ESCOP 1997).

(66) McGuffin M, Hobbs C, Upton R, Goldberg A (eds.). *American Herbal Products Association's Botanical Safety Handbook.* 1st ed., (Boca Raton, FL: CRC Press. 1997).

(67) SC Piscitelli et al. The effect of garlic supplements on the pharmacokinetics of saquinavir. "Clinical Infectious Diseases" Electronic Edition (December 3, 2001)

Chapter 17 - Propolis References

(1) Sangvai S, Chianese J, Morone N, Bogen DL, Voigt L, Shaikh N. Can an herbal preparation of echinacea, propolis, and vitamin C reduce respiratory illnesses in children? Arch Pediatr Adolesc Med. 2004 Mar;158(3):222-4.

(2) Hegazi AG, Abd El Hady FK. Egyptian propolis. Antioxidant, antimicrobial activities and chemical composition of propolis from reclaimed lands. Z Naturforsch [C]. 2002 Mar-Apr;57(3-4):395-402.

(3) Hill R. Propolis, The Natural Antibiotic. Thorsons, Wellingborough, England, 1977.

(4) Tsarev NI, Petrik EV, Aleksandrova VI. Use of propolis in the treatment of local suppurative infection. Vestn Khir, 134 (5): 119-122, 1985.

(5) Esanu V. Recent Advances in the chemotherapy of herpes virus infections. Virologie, 32 (1): 57-77, 1981.

(6) Pang JF and Chen SS. Treatment of oral leukoplakia with propolis: Report of 45 cases. Chung Hsi I Chieh Ho Tsa Chih, 5 (8): 452-453 and 485-486, 1985.

(7) Kravcuk P. Doctoral Dissertation. Kiev Univ., USSR, 1971.

(8) Serkedjieva J, Manolova N, and Bankova V. Anti-influenza virus effect of some propolis constituents and their analogues (esters of substituted cinnamic acids). J. Natl. Prod., 55 (3): 294-302, 1992.

(9) Amoros M, Lurton E, Boustie J, Girre L, Sauvager F, and Cormier M. Comparison of the anti-herpes simplex virus activities of propolis and 3-methyl -but-2-enyl caffeate. J. Natl. Prod., 57 (5): 644-647, 1994.

(10) Dumitrescu M, E sanu, and Cri san I. The mechanisms of the antiherpetic action of aqueous propolis extracts. I. The antioxidant action on human fibroblast cultures. Rev. Roum. Virol., 43: 3-4 and 165-173, 1992.

(11) Takaisi-Kikuni NB and Schilcher H. Electron microscopic and microcalorimetric investigations of the possible mechanism of the antibacterial action of a defined propolis provenance. Planta Med., 60 (3): 222-227, 1994.

(12) Krol W, Schelleer S, Shani J, Pietsz G, and Czuba Z. Synergistic effect of ethanolic extract of propolis and antibiotics on the growth of staphylococcus aureus. Arzneimittelforschung, 43 (5): 607-609, 1993.

(13) Churchill R. American Chiropractor, 34-38, January/February 1980.

(14) Dim V, Ivanovska N, Bankova V, and Popov S. Immunomodulatory action of propolis: IV. Prophylactic activity against gram-negative infections and adjuvant effect of the water-soluble derivative. Vaccine, 10 (12): 817-823, 1992.

138

(15) Sudina GF, Mirzoeva OK, Pushkareva MA, Korshunova GA, Sumbatyan NV, and Varfolomeev SD. Caffeic acid phenethyl ester as a lipoxygenase inhibitor with antioxidant properties. FEBS Lett., 329: 1-2, 21-24, 1993.

(16) Strehl E, Volpert R, and Elstner EF. Biochemical activities of propolis - extracts. III. Inhibition of dihydrofolate reductase. Z Naturfosch [C], 49: 1-2, 39 -43, 1994.

(17) Rao CV, Desai D, Kaul B, Amin S, and Reddy BS. Effect of caffeic acid esters on carcinogen-induced mutagenicity and human colon adenocarcinoma cell growth. Chem. Biol. Interact., 84 (3): 277-90, 1992.

(18) Rao CV, Desai D, Rivenson A, Simi B, Amin S, and Reddy BS. Chemoprevention of colon carcinogenesis by phenylethyl-3-methylcaffeate. Cancer Res., 55 (11): 2310-2315, 1995.

(19) Guarini L, Su ZZ, Zucker S, Lin J, Grunberger D, and Fisher PB. Growth inhibition and modulation of antigenic phenotype in human melanoma and glioblastoma multiform cells by caffecic acid phenethyl ester (CAPE). Cell Mol. Biol., 38 (5): 513-527, 1992.

(20) Su ZZ, Lin J, Prewett M, Goldstein NI, and Fisher PB. Apoptosis www.es the selective toxicity of caffeic acid phenethyl ester (CAPE) toward oncogene - transformed rat embryo fibroblast cells. Anticancer Res., 15 (5B): 1841-1848, 1995.

(21) Chiao C, Carothers AM, Grunberger D, Solomon G, Preston GA, and Barrett JC. Apoptosis and altered redox state induced by caffeic acid phenethyl ester (CAPE) in transformed rat fibroblast cells. Cancer Res., 55 (16): 3576-3583, 1995.

(22) Chopra S, Pillai KK, Husain SZ, and Giri DK. Propolis protects against doxorubicin-induced myocardiopathy in rats. Exp. Mol. Pathol., 62 (3): 190-198, 1995.

(23) Brätter, C.; Tregel M., Liebenthal C., Volk H. D. (October 1999). "Prophylactic effectiveness of propolis for immunostimulation: a clinical pilot study". Forsch Komplementarmed. 6 (5): 256-60.

(24) Arvouet-Grand A, Lejeune B, Bastide P, Pourrat A, Privat AM, and Legret P. Propolis extract. I. Acute toxicity and determination of acute primary cutaneous irritation index. J. Pharm. Belg., 48 (3): 165-170, 1993.

(25) Huleihel M, Isanu V. Anti-herpes simplex virus effect of an aqueous extract of propolis. Isr Med Assoc J. 2002 Nov;4(11 Suppl):923-7.

(26) Dumitrescu M, E sanu, and Cri san I. The mechanisms of the antiherpetic action of aqueous propolis extracts. I. The antioxidant action on human fibroblast cultures. Rev. Roum. Virol., 43: 3-4 and 165-173, 1992.

(27) Gregory, S. R.; Piccolo N., Piccolo M. T., Piccolo M. S., Heggers J. P. (February 2002). "Abstract Comparison of propolis skin cream to silver sulfadiazine: a naturopathic alternative to antibiotics in treatment of minor burns". J Altern Complement Med. 8 (1): 77-83.

139

(28) Hoşnuter, M.; Gürel A., Babucçu O., Armutcu F., Kargi E., Işikdemir A. (March 2004). "The effect of CAPE on lipid peroxidation and nitric oxide levels in the plasma of rats following thermal injury". *Burns* **30** (2): 121-5.

(29) Ocakci, A.; Kanter M., Cabuk M., Buyukbas S. (October 2006). "Role of caffeic acid phenethyl ester, an active component of propolis, against NAOH-induced esophageal burns in rats". *Int J Pediatr Otorhinolaryngol.* **70** (10): 1731-9.

(30) Ansorge, S.; Reinhold D., Lendeckel U. (July-August 2003). "Propolis and some of its constituents down-regulate DNA synthesis and inflammatory cytokine production but induce TGF-beta1 production of human immune cells". *Z Naturforsch [C].* **58** (7-8): 580-9.

(31) Botushanov, P. I.; Grigorov G. I., Aleksandrov G. A. (2001). "A clinical study of a silicate toothpaste with extract from propolis". *Folia Med (Plovdiv)* **43** (1-2): 28-30.

(32) Koo, H.; Cury J. A., Rosalen P. L., Ambrosano G. M., Ikegaki M., Park Y. K. (November-December 2002). "Effect of a mouthrinse containing selected propolis on 3-day dental plaque accumulation and polysaccharide formation". *Caries Research* **36** (6): 445-8.

(33) Duarte, S.; Rosalen P. L., Hayacibara M. F., Cury J. A., Bowen W. H., Marquis R. E., Rehder V. L., Sartoratto A., Ikegaki M., Koo H. (January 2006). "The influence of a novel propolis on mutans streptococci biofilms and caries development in rats". *Arch Oral Biol.* **51** (1): 15-22.

(34) Park, Y. K.; Koo M. H., Abreu J. A., Ikegaki M., Cury J. A., Rosalen P. L. (January 1998). "Antimicrobial activity of propolis on oral microorganisms". *Curr Microbiol.* **36** (1): 24-8.

Chapter 18 - Oral Proteolytic Enzyme References

(1) Brendel R, Beiler JM, Martin GJ. *American Journal of Pharmacology* 1956;128:172.

(2) Martin GJ, Brendal R, Beiler JM. Uptake of labelled chymotrypsin across the GI. *American Journal of Pharmacology* 1957;129:194-197.

(3) Ambrus JC, Lassman HB, Marchijj DE. Absorption of exogenous and endogenous proteolytic enzymes. *Clinical Pharmacology and Therapeutics* 1967;8(3):362-367.

(4) Vakians A. Further studies on the absorption of chymotrypsin. *Clinical Pharmacology and Therapeutics* 1964:5(6):712-715.

(5) Miller J, Opher A. Increased proteolytic activity of human blood serum after oral administration of bromelain. *Exp Med Surg* 1964;22:277.

(6) Innerfield I, Wernick T. Plasma anti-thrombin alterations following oral papain. *Proc Soc Ext Biol Med* July 1961;107:505-506.

(7) Miller J. Absorption of proteolytic enzymes from the gastrointestinal tract. *Clinical Medicine* October 1968;75:35-40.

(8) Ito C. Anti-inflammatory actions of proteases, bromelain, trypsin and their mixed preparations. *Folia Pharmacol JPN* 1979;75:227.

(9) Kabacoff B, Wohlman A, et al. Absorption of chymotrypsin from the intestinal tract. *Nature* 1963;199:815.

(10) Taussig SJ, Batkin S. Bromelain, the enzyme complex of pineapple (*Ananas comosus*) and its clinical application.. An update. *J Ethnopharmacol.* 1988;22:191-203

(11) Deitrick RE. Oral Proteolytic Enzymes in the treatment of athletic injuries: a double-blind study. *Pa Med.* 1965;68:35–37

(12) Blonstein JL. Control of swelling in boxing injuries. *Practitioner.* 1969;203:206.

(13) Baumuller M. The application of hydrolytic enzymes in blunt wounds to the soft tissue and distortion of the
ankle joint: a double-blind clinical trial [translated from German]. *Allgemeinmedizin.* 1990;19:178–182.

(14) Zuschlag JM. Double-blind clinical study using certain pproteolytic enzyme mixtures in karate fighters. Working paper. *Mucos Pharma GmbH (Germany).* 1988;1–5.

(15) Rathgeber WF. The use of proteolytic enzymes (Chymoral) in sporting injuries. *S Afr Med J.* 1971;45:181–183.

(16) Deitrick RE. Oral Proteolytic Enzymes in the treatment of athletic injuries: a double-blind study. *Pa Med.* 1965;68:35–37

(17) Smyth RD, Brennan R, Martin GJ. Studies establishing the absorption of bromelains (Proteolytic enzymes) from the gastrointestinal tract. *Exp Med Surg.* 1964;22: 46–59.

(18) Miller JM, Ginseberg M, McElfatrick GC, et al. The administration of bromelain orally in the treatment of inflammation and edema. *Exp Med Surg.* 1964;22:293–299.

(19) Castell JV, Friedrich G, Kuhn CS, et al. Intestinal absorption of undegraded proteins in men: presence of bromelain in plasma after oral intake. *Am J Physiol.* 1997;273:G139–G146.

(20) Billigmann VP. Enzyme therapy—an alternative in treatment of herpes zoster. A controlled study of 192 patients [translated from German]. *Fortschr Med.* 1995;113:43–48.

(21) Kleine MW, Stauder GM, Beese EW. The intestinal absorption of orally administered hydrolytic enzymes and their effects in the treatment of acute

herpes zoster as compared with those of oral acyclovir therapy. *Phytomedicine.* 1995;2:7–15.

(22) Baumuller M. The application of hydrolytic enzymes in blunt wounds to the soft tissue and distortion of the ankle joint: a double-blind clinical trial [translated from German]. *Allgemeinmedizin.* 1990;19:178–182.

(23) Zuschlag JM. Double-blind clinical study using certain proteolytic enzyme mixtures in karate fighters. Working paper. *Mucos Pharma GmbH (Germany).* 1988;1–5.

(24) Rathgeber WF. The use of proteolytic enzymes (Chymoral) in sporting injuries. *S Afr Med J.* 1971;45:181–183.

(25) Deitrick RE. Oral Proteolytic Enzymes in the treatment of athletic injuries: a double-blind study. *Pa Med.*1965;68:35–37.

(26) Shaw PC. The use of a trypsin-chymotrypsin formulation in fractures of the hand. *Br J Clin Pract.* 1969;23:25–26.

(27) Kleine MW, Pabst H. The effect of an oral enzyme therapy on experimentally produced hematomas [translated from German]. *Forum des Prakt und Allgemeinarztes.* 1988;27:42, 45–46, 48.

(28) Rahn HD. Efficacy of hydrolytic enzymes in surgery. Paper presented at: 24th FIMS World Congress of Sports Medicine; May 27-June 1, 1990; Amsterdam.

(29) Vinzenz K. Treatment of edema with hydrolytic enzymes in oral surgical procedures [translated from German]. *Quintessenz.* 1991;42:1053–1064.

(30) Seltzer AP. Minimizing post-operative edema and ecchymoses by the use of an oral enzyme preparation (bromelain): a controlled study of 53 rhinoplasty cases. *Eye Ear Nose Throat Mon.* 1962;41:813–817.

(31) Blonstein JL. Control of swelling in boxing injuries. *Practitioner.* 1969;203:206. 26. Zatuchni GI, Colombi DJ. Bromelains therapy for the prevention of episiotomy pain. *Obstet Gynecol.* 1967;29:275–278.

(32) Zatuchni GI, Colombi DJ. Bromelains therapy for the prevention of episiotomy pain. *Obstet Gynecol.* 1967;29:275-278.

(33) Spaeth GL. The effect of bromelains on the inflammatory response caused by cataract extraction: a double-blind study. *Eye Ear Nose Throat Mon.* 1968;47:634–639.

(34) Tassman GC, Zafran JN, Zayon GM. Evaluation of a plant proteolytic enzyme for the control of imflammation and pain. *J Dent Med.* 1964;19:73–77.

(35) Howat RC, Lewis GD. The effect of bromelain therapy on episiotomy wounds—a double-blind controlled clinical trial. *J Obstet Gynaecol Br Commonw.* 1972;79:951–953.

142

(36) Gylling U, Rintala A, Taipale S, et al. The effect of a proteolytic enzyme combinate (bromelain) on the postoperative oedema by oral application. A clinical and experimental study. *Acta Chir Scand.*1966;131:193–196.

(37) Cameron IW. An investigation into some of the factors concerned in the surgical removal of the impacted lower wisdom tooth, including a double blind trial of chymoral. *Br J Oral Surg.* 1980;18:112–124.

(38) Soule SD, Wasserman HC, Burstein R. Oral Proteolytic enzyme therapy (Chymoral) in episiotomy patients. *Am J Obstet Gynecol.* 1966;95:820–823.

(40) Howat RC, Lewis GD. The effect of bromelain therapy on episiotomy wounds—a double blind controlled clinical trial. *J Obstet Gynaecol Br Commow.* 1972;79:951–953.

(41) Frank SC. Use of chymoral as an anti-inflammatory agent following surgical trauma. *J Am Podiatr Assoc.*1965;55:706–709.

(42) Gylling U, Rintala A, Taipale S, et al. The effect of a proteolytic enzyme combinate (bromelain) on the postoperative oedema by oral application. A clinical and experimental study. *Acta Chir Scand.*1966;131:193–196.

(43) Tilscher H, Keusch R, Neumann K. Results of a double-blind, randomized comparative study of WobenzymW-placebo in patients with cervical syndrome [translated from German]. *Wien Med Wochenschr* .1996;146:91-95.

(44) Singer F, Oberleitner H. Drug therapy of activated arthrosis. On the effectiveness of an enzyme mixture versus DiclofenacW [translated from German]. *Wien Med Wochenschr* . 1996;146:55-58.

(45) Klein G, Kullich W. Reducing pain by oral enzyme therapy in rheumatic diseases [translated from German]. *Wien Med Wochenschr* . 1999;149:577-580.

(46) Russell RM, Dutta SK, Oaks EV, et al. Impairment of folic acid absorption by oral pancreatic extracts. *DigDis Sci.* 1980;25:369–373.

(47) Shaw D, Leon C, Kolev S, et al. Traditional remedies and food supplements. A 5-year toxicological study (1991-1995). *Drug Saf.* 1997;17:342–356.

(48) Layer P, Groger G. Fate of pancreatic enzymes in the human intestinal lumen in health and pancreatic insufficiency. *Digestion* 1993;54(suppl 2):10–4.

(49) Hingorani K. Oral enzyme therapy in severe back pain. *Br J Clin Pract* 1968;22:209–10.

(50) Gaspardy G, Balint G, Mitsuova M, et al. Treatment of sciatica due to intervertebral disc herniation with Chymoral tablets. *Rheum Phys Med* 1971;11:14–9.

(51) Stevens JC, Maguiness KM, Hollingsworth J, et al. Pancreatic enzyme supplementation in cystic fibrosis patients before and after fibrosing colonopathy. *J Pediatr Gastroenterol Nutr* 1998;26:80–4.

(52) Oades PJ, Bush A, Ong PS, Brereton RJ. High-strength pancreatic enzyme supplements and large-bowel stricture in cystic fibrosis. *Lancet* 1994;343:109 [letter].

(53) Campbell CA, Forrest J, Muscgrove C. High-strength pancreatic enzyme supplements and large-bowel stricture in cystic fibrosis. *Lancet* 1994;343:109–10 [letter].

(54) Milla CE, Wielinski CL, Warwick WJ. High-strength pancreatic enzymes. *Lancet* 1994;343:599 [letter].

(55) Jones R, Franklin K, Spicer R, Berry J. Colonic strictures in children with cystic fibrosis on low-strength pancreatic enzymes. *Lancet* 1995;346:499–500 [letter].

(56) Powell CJ. Pancreatic enzymes and fibrosing colonopathy. *Lancet* 1999;354:251 [letter].

(57) Clinical Experience with Systemic Enzyme Therapy in the Treatment of Herpes zoster, Pospíšilová A., Haklová L. II. dermato-venerology clinic, Faculty Hospital Brno-Bohunice Cesko-slovenská dermatologie, 1999, 74 (1), 17-20.

(58) Possibility to Treat Herpes zoster Using Enzymes I. Mikazans Department of Dermatology, Medical Academy of Latvia, Riga, Latvia Australasian Journal of Dermatology 38 (2), 1997. Abstracts of the 19th World Congress of Dermatology, 15-20 June, 1997, Sydney, Australia

(59) Introduction to Oral Enzyme Therapy and Its Use in Varicella zoster Treatment Kleine M.-W., Ertl D. Allergist, Egenhofenstrasse 18, 82152 Planegg/Munich, Germany Int J Tiss Reac XIX (1/2), 1997 - abstracts of 7th Interscience World Conference on Inflammation, Antirheumatics, Analgesics, Immunomodulators, May 19-21, Geneva, Switzerland

(60) Hydrolytic Enzymes in the Treatment of HIV Infections H. Jäger. Allgemeinmedizin (1990) 19: 160-164 Kuratorium für Immunschwäche, München.

(61) Oral Enzyme Therapy in Hepatitis C patients Stauder G.,1 Kabil S.2. Int. J. Immunotherapy XIII(3/4) 153-158 (1997).

(62) Clinical use of Belosorb and Wobenzym in the Treatment of Viral Hepatitis B Nikolaev V.G., Matiasch V.I., Kononenko V.V. Kiev, Ukraine. Presented at the conference "Current approaches in infectology, epidemiology, and microbiology", Kiev, 1998.

(63) A Study of Serum Glycolytic Enzymes and Serum B Hepatitis in Relation to LIV.52 Therapy Patney NL, Pachori S. The Medicine and Surgery 1986;4:9

(64) Stauder G, Kabil S. Oral enzyme therapy in hepatitis C patients. Int J Immunother 1997;3:153-158 Kabil S, Stauder G. Oral enzyme therapy in hepatitis C patients. Int J Tiss Reac 1997;1-2

(65) Gonzalez NJ, Isaacs LL: Evaluation of pancreatic proteolytic enzyme treatment of adenocarcinoma of the pancreas, with nutrition and detoxification support. Nutr Cancer 1999;33:117-24.

(66) Leipner J, Saller R: Systemic enzyme therapy in oncology: effect and mode of action. Drugs. 2000;59:769-80.

(67) Murray Michael. Proteolytic enzymes in the treatment of acute herpes zoster. The American Journal of Natural Medicine. 1996;17.

(68) Murray Michael. Encyclopedia of Nutritional Supplements.1996.

(69) Murray Michael. The Healing Power of Proteolytic Enzymes.2004

Chapter 19 - Indole-3 Carbinol References

(1) Michnovicz JJ, Bradlow HL. Induction of estradiol metabolism by dietary indole-3-carbinol in humans. *J Natl Cancer Inst*. 1990; 50:947-950.

(2) Stoner TD, Sweet TJ, Fu MM, Delucia AL, Docherty JJ. Indole-3-Carbinol Inhibits Herpes Simplex Virus Replication. Interscience Conference on Antimicrobial Agents and Chemotherapy, presentation number V-287. Cruciferous Vegetables and Breast Cancer Risk: Results from the US Component of the Polish Women's Health Study (PWHS)

(3) http://www.ihcs.msu.edu/Obesity/Nutrigenomics/DP-Cabbage-sauerkraut-MSU-11-4-05.pdf. Stoewsand GS. Bioactive organosulfur phytochemicals in Brassica oleracea vegetables—a review. *Food Chem Toxicol* 1995;33:537–43.

(4) Broadbent TA, Broadbent HS. The chemistry and pharmacology of indole-3-carbinol (indole-3-methanol) and 3-(methoxymethyl)indole. [Part I]. *Curr Med Chem* 1998;5:337–52.

(5) Broadbent TA, Broadbent HS. The chemistry and pharmacology of indole-3-carbinol (indole-3-methanol) and 3-(methoxymethyl)indole. [Part II]. *Curr Med Chem* 1998;5:469–91.

(6) Albert-Puleo M. Physiological effects of cabbage with reference to its potential as a dietary cancer-inhibitor and its use in ancient medicine. *J Ethnopharm*. 1983; 9:261-272.

(7) Osborne MP, Bradlow HL, Wong GY, Telang NT. Upregulation of estradiol C16 alpha-hydroxylation in human breast tissue: a potential biomarker of breast cancer risk. J National Cancer Inst 1993; 85(23): 1917-1920.

(8) Michnoviez JJ, Bradlow HL. Altered estrogen metabolism and excretion in humans following consumption of indole-3-carbinol. Nutr Cancer 1991;16 (1): 59-66.

(9) Michnoviez JJ, Bradlow HL. Induction of estradiol metabolism by dietary indole-3-carbinol in humans. J Natl Cancer Inst. 1990; 82(11): 947-949.

(10) Fahey JW, Zalcmann AT, Talalay P. The chemical diversity and distribution of glucosinolates and isothiocyanates among plants. Phytochemistry. 2001;56(1):5-51

(11) Chen DZ, Qi M, Auborn KJ, Carter TH. Indole-3-carbinol and diindolylmethane induce apoptosis of human cervical cancer cells and in murine HPV16-transgenic preneoplastic cervical epithelium. J Nutr 2001 Dec;131(12):3294-302.

(12) McAlindon TE, Gulin J, Chen T, Klug T, Lahita R, Nuite M. Indole-3-carbinol in women with SLE: effect on estrogen metabolism and disease activity. Lupus 2001;10(11):779-83.

(13) Auborn KJ, Qi M, Yan XJ, Teichberg S, Chen D, Madaio MP, Chiorazzi N. Lifespan is prolonged in autoimmune-prone (NZB/NZW) F1 mice fed a diet supplemented with indole-3-carbinol. J Nutr 2003 Nov;133(11):3610-3.

(14) He YH, Friesen MD, Ruch RJ, Schut HA. Indole-3-carbinol as a chemopreventive agent in 2-amino-1-methyl-6-phenylimidazo[4,5-b]pyridine (PhIP) carcinogenesis: inhibition of PhIP-DNA adduct formation, acceleration of PhIP metabolism, and induction of cytochrome P450 in female F344 rats. Food Chem Toxicol. 2000;38(1):15-23.

(15) Lake BG, Tredger JM, Renwick AB, Barton PT, Price RJ. 3,3'-Diindolylmethane induces CYP1A2 in cultured precision-cut human liver slices. Xenobiotica. 1998;28(8):803-811.

(16) Leibelt DA, Hedstrom OR, Fischer KA, Pereira CB, Williams DE. Evaluation of chronic dietary exposure to indole-3-carbinol and absorption-enhanced 3,3'-diindolylmethane in sprague-dawley rats. Toxicol Sci. 2003;74(1):10-21.

(17) Dashwood RH. Indole-3-carbinol: anticarcinogen or tumor promoter in brassica vegetables? *Chem Biol Interact*. 1998;110:1–5.
(18) Bailey GS, Hendricks JD, Shelton DW, et al. Enhancement of carcinogenesis by the natural anticarcinogen indole-3-carbinol. *J Natl Cancer Inst*. 1987;78:931–934.

(19) Meng Q, Yuan F, Goldberg ID, et al. Indole-3-carbinol is a negative regulator of estrogen receptor-alpha signaling in human tumor cells. *J Nutr.* 2000;130:2927-293l.

(20) Wong GY, Bradlow L, Sepkovic D, Mehl S, Mailman J, Osborne MP. Dose-ranging study of indole-3-carbinol for breast cancer prevention. J Cell Biochem Suppl. 1997;28-29:111-116.

(21) McAlindon TE, Gulin J, Chen T, Klug T, Lahita R, Nuite M. Indole-3-carbinol in women with SLE: effect on estrogen metabolism and disease activity. Lupus. 2001;10(11):779-783.

146

(22) Rosen CA, Woodson GE, Thompson JW, Hengesteg AP, Bradlow HL. Preliminary results of the use of indole-3-carbinol for recurrent respiratory papillomatosis. Otolaryngol Head Neck Surg. 1998;118(6):810-815.

(23) Stoner G, Casto B, Ralston S, Roebuck B, Pereira C, Bailey G. Development of a multi-organ rat model for evaluating chemopreventive agents: efficacy of indole-3-carbinol. Carcinogenesis. 2002;23(2):265-272.

(24) Pence BC, Buddingh F, Yang SP. Multiple dietary factors in the enhancement of dimethylhydrazine carcinogenesis: main effect of indole-3-carbinol. J Natl Cancer Inst. 1986;77(1):269-276.

(25) Yoshida M, Katashima S, Ando J, et al. Dietary indole-3-carbinol promotes endometrial adenocarcinoma development in rats initiated with N-ethyl-N'-nitro-N-nitrosoguanidine, with induction of cytochrome P450s in the liver and consequent modulation of estrogen metabolism. Carcinogenesis. 2004;25(11):2257-2264.

(26) Kim DJ, Han BS, Ahn B, et al. Enhancement by indole-3-carbinol of liver and thyroid gland neoplastic development in a rat medium-term multiorgan carcinogenesis model. Carcinogenesis. 1997;18(2):377-381.

(27) Wong GY, Bradlow L, Sepkovic D, Mehl S, Mailman J, Osborne MP. Dose-ranging study of indole-3-carbinol for breast cancer prevention. J Cell Biochem Suppl. 1997;28-29:111-116.

(28) Rosen CA, Woodson GE, Thompson JW, Hengesteg AP, Bradlow HL. Preliminary results of the use of indole-3-carbinol for recurrent respiratory papillomatosis. Otolaryngol Head Neck Surg. 1998;118(6):810-815.

(29) Rosen CA, Bryson PC. Indole-3-carbinol for recurrent respiratory papillomatosis: long-term results. J Voice. 2004;18(2):248-253.

(30) Dalessandri KM, Firestone GL, Fitch MD, Bradlow HL, Bjeldanes LF. Pilot study: effect of 3,3'-diindolylmethane supplements on urinary hormone metabolites in postmenopausal women with a history of early-stage breast cancer. Nutr Cancer. 2004;50(2):161-167.

Chapter 20 - Resveratrol References

(1) Avellone G, Di Garbo V, Campisi D, De Simone R, Raneli G, Scaglione R, Licata G. Effects of moderate Sicilian red wine consumption on inflammatory biomarkers of atherosclerosis. Eur J Clin Nutr. 2006; 60:41-7.

(2) Anekonda TS. Resveratrol-a boon for treating Alzheimer's disease? Brain Res Brain Res Rev. 2006 Sep;52(2):316-26.

(3) Aggarwal BB, Bhardwaj A, Aggarwal RS, et al. Role of resveratrol in prevention and therapy of cancer: preclinical and clinical studies. Anticancer Res. 2004 Sep;24(5A):2783-840.

(4) Baur JA, Pearson KJ, Price NL, et al. Resveratrol improves health and survival of mice on a high-calorie diet. Nature. 2006 Nov 16;444(7117):337-42.

(5) Bauer JH, Goupil S, Garber GB, Helfand SL. An accelerated assay for the identification of lifespan-extending interventions in Drosophila melanogaster. Proc Natl Acad Sci U S A. 2004 Aug 31;101(35):12980-5.

(6) Zou J, Huang Y, Chen Q, et al. Suppression of mitogenesis and regulation of cell cycle traverse by resveratrol in cultured smooth muscle cells. Int J Oncol. 1999; 15:647-651.

(7) Bhat KPL, Kosmeder JW, Pezzuto JM. Biological effects of resveratrol. Antioxid Redox Signal. 2001 Dec;3(6):1041-64.

(8) Borra MT, Smith BC, Denu JM. Mechanism of human SIRT1 activation by resveratrol. J Biol Chem. 2005 Apr 29;280(17):17187-95.

(9) Bowers JL, Tyulmenkov VV, Jernigan SC, Klinge CM. Resveratrol acts as a mixed agonist/antagonist for estrogen receptors alpha and beta. Endocrinology. 2000; 141:3657-3667.

(10) Brito PM, Mariano A, Almeida LM, Dinis TC. Resveratrol affords protection against peroxynitrite-mediated endothelial cell death: A role for intracellular glutathione. Chem Biol Interact. 2006 Dec 15;164(3):157-66.

(11) Bujanda L, Garcia-Barcina M, Gutierrez-de JV, et al. Effect of resveratrol on alcohol-induced mortality and liver lesions in mice. BMC Gastroenterol. 2006 Nov 14;6:35.

(12) Burkitt MJ, Duncan J. Effects of trans-resveratrol on copper-dependent hydroxyl-radical formation and DNA damage: Evidence for hydroxyl-radical scavenging and a novel. Glutathione-sparing mechanism of action. Arch Biochem Biophys. 2000; 381:253-263.

(13) Cao G, Prior RL. Red wine in moderation: Potential health benefits independent of alcohol. Nutr Clin Care. 2000; 3:76-82.

(14) Chen WP, Su MJ, Hung LM. In vitro electrophysiological mechanisms for antiarrhythmic efficacy of resveratrol, a red wine antioxidant. Eur J Pharmacol. 2007 Jan 12;554(2-3):196-204.

(15) Chun YJ, Kim MY, Guengerich FP. Resveratrol is a selective human cytochrome P450 1A1 inhibitor. Biochem Biophys Res Commun. 1999; 262:20-24.

(16) Cichewicz RH, Kouzi SA, Hamann MT. Dimerization of resveratrol by the grapevine pathogen. Botrytis cinerea. J Natl Prod. 2000; 63:29-33.

(17) Ciolino HP, Yeh GC. Inhibition of aryl hydrocarbon-induced cytochrome P450 1A1 enzyme activity and CYP1A1 expression by resveratrol. Mol Pharmacol. 1999; 56:760-767.

148

(18) Constant J. Alcohol, ischemic heart disease, and the French paradox. Coron Artery Dis. 1997 Oct;8(10):645-9.

(19) De Santi C, Pietrabissa A, Spisni R, Mosca F, Pacifici GM. Sulphation of resveratrol, a natural compound present in wine, and its inhibition by natural flavonoids. Xenobiotica. 2000 Sep;30(9):857-66.

(20) De Santi C, Pietrabissa A, Spisni R, Mosca F, Pacifici GM. Sulphation of resveratrol, a natural product present in grapes and wine, in the human liver and duodenum. Xenobiotica. 2000 Jun;30(6):609-17.

(21) Docherty JJ, Smith JS, Fu MM, Stoner T, Booth T. Effect of topically applied resveratrol on cutaneous herpes simplex virus infection in hairless mice. Antiviral Res 2004;61:19-26.

(22) Docherty JJ, Fu MM, Hah JM, Sweet TJ, Faith SA, Booth T. Effect of resveratrol on herpes simplex virus vaginal infection in the mouse. Antiviral Res 2005;67:155-62.

(23) Docherty JJ, Fu MM, Stiffer BS, et al. Resveratrol inhibition of herpes simplex virus replication. Antiviral Res. 1999; 43:145-155.
(24) Dong Z. Molecular mechanism of the chemopreventive effect of resveratrol. Mutat Res. 2003 Feb;523-524:145-50.

(25) Dubash BD, Zheng BL, Kim CH, et al. Inhibitory effect of resveratrol and related compounds on the macromolecular synthesis in HL-60 cells and the metabolism of 7,12-dimethylbenz[a]anthracene by mouse liver microsomes. In: Shahidi F, Ho C-T, eds. Phytochemicals and Phytopharmaceuticals. Champaign, IL: AOCS Press; 2000:314-320.

(26) Dye D. Grape seed blocks colon cancer cell growth. Life Extension. January, 2007:13.

(27) Elmali N, Baysal O, Harma A, Esenkaya I, Mizrak B. Effects of resveratrol in inflammatory arthritis. Inflammation. 2006 Nov 4.

(28) Folts JD. Potential health benefits from the flavonoids in grape products on vascular disease. Adv Exp Med Biol. 2002;505:95-111.

(29) Fontecave M, Lepoivre M, Elleingand E, et al. Resveratrol, a remarkable inhibitor of ribonucleotide reductase. FEBS Lett. 1998; 421:277-279.

(30) Fremont L. Biological effects of resveratrol. Life Sci. 2000 Jan 14;66(8):663-73.

(31) Frémont L, Belguendouz L, Delpal S. Antioxidant activity of resveratrol and alcohol-free wine polyphenols related to LDL oxidation and polyunsaturated fatty acids. Life Sci. 1999; 64:2511-2521.

(32) Gehm BD, McAndrews JM, Chien P-Y, Jameson JL. Resveratrol, a polyphenolic compound found in grapes and wine, is an agonist for the estrogen receptor. Proc Natl Acad Sci USA. 1997; 94:14138-14143.

(33) Goh SS, Woodman OL, Pepe S, et al. The red wine antioxidant resveratrol prevents cardiomyocyte injury following ischemia-reperfusion via multiple sites and mechanisms. Antioxid Redox Signal. 2007 Jan;9(1):101-13.

(34) Guarente L, Picard F. Calorie restriction-the SIR2 connection. Cell. 2005 Feb 25;120(4):473-82.

(35) Halioua B, Malkin JE. Epidemiology of genital herpes-recent advances. Eur J Dermatol 1999;9:177-84

(36) Harper JM, Salmon AB, Chang Y, et al. Stress resistance and aging: influence of genes and nutrition. Mech Ageing Dev. 2006 Aug;127(8):687-94.

(37) Hayashi A, Gillen AC, Lott JR. Effects of daily oral administration of quercetin chalcone and modified citrus pectin on implanted colon-25 tumor growth in Balb-c mice. Altern Med Rev. 2000 Dec;5(6):546-52.

(38) Heilbronn LK, de Jonge L, Frisard MI, et al. Effect of 6-month calorie restriction on biomarkers of longevity, metabolic adaptation, and oxidative stress in overweight individuals: a randomized controlled trial. JAMA. 2006 Apr 5;295(13):1539-48.

(39) Holmes-McNary M, Baldwin AS Jr. Chemopreventive properties of trans-resveratrol are associated with inhibition of activation of the IkappaB kinase. Cancer Res. 2000; 60:3477-3483.

(40) Hsieh TC, Juan G, Darzynkiewicz Z, Wu JM. Resveratrol increases nitric oxide synthase, induces accumulation of p53 and p21 (WAF1/CIP1), and suppresses cultured bovine pulmonary artery endothelial cell proliferation by perturbing progression through S and G2. Cancer Res. 1999; 59:2596-2601.

(41) Hung L-M, Chen J-K, Huang S-S, et al. Cardioprotective effect of resveratrol, a natural antioxidant derived from grapes. Cardiovascular Res. 2000; 47:549-555.

(42) Heynekamp JJ, Weber WM, Hunsaker LA, et al. Substituted trans-stilbenes, including analogues of the natural product resveratrol, inhibit the human tumor necrosis factor alpha-induced activation of transcription factor nuclear factor KappaB. J Med Chem. 2006 Nov 30;49(24):7182-9.

(45) Ignatowicz E, Baer-Dubowska W. Resveratrol, a natural chemopreventive agent against degenerative diseases. Pol J Pharmacol. 2001 Nov;53(6):557-69.

(46) Ingram DK, Anson RM, de Cabo R, et al. Development of calorie restriction mimetics as a prolongevity strategy. Ann NY Acad Sci. 2004 Jun;1019:412-23.

(47) Ingram DK, Zhu M, Mamczarz J, et al. Calorie restriction mimetics: an emerging research field. Aging Cell. 2006 Apr;5(2):97-108.

(48) Jang M, Cai L, Udeani GO, et al. Cancer chemopreventive activity of resveratrol, a natural product derived from grapes. Science. 1997; 275:218-220.

150

(49) Jang M, Pezzuto JM. Cancer chemopreventive activity of resveratrol. Drugs Exp Clin Res. 1999; 25:65-77.

(50) Kaeberlein M, McDonagh T, Heltweg B, et al. Substrate-specific activation of sirtuins by resveratrol. J Biol Chem. 2005 Apr 29;280(17):17038-45.

(51) Kiefer D. Preserving and restoring brain function. Life Extension. October, 2005:36-45.

(52) Kim H, Deshane J, Barnes S, Meleth S. Proteomics analysis of the actions of grape seed extract in rat brain: technological and biological implications for the study of the actions of psychoactive compounds. Life Sci. 2006 Mar 27;78(18):2060-5.

(53) Kirk RI, Deitch JA, Wu JM, Lerea KM. Resveratrol decreases early signaling events in washed platelets but has little effect on platelet aggregation in whole blood. Blood Cells Mol Dis. 2000; 26:144-150.

(54) Kumar P, Padi SS, Naidu PS, Kumar A. Effect of resveratrol on 3-nitropropionic acid-induced biochemical and behavioural changes: possible neuroprotective mechanisms. Behav Pharmacol. 2006 Sep;17(5-6):485-92.

(55) Lagouge M, Argmann C, Gerhart-Hines Z, et al. Resveratrol improves mitochondrial function and protects against metabolic disease by activating SIRT1 and PGC-1alpha. Cell. 2006 Dec 15;127(6):1109-22.

(56) Luo L, Huang YM. Effect of resveratrol on the cognitive ability of Alzheimer's mice. Zhong Nan Da Xue Xue Bao Yi Xue Ban. 2006 Aug;31(4):566-9.

(57) Marambaud P, Zhao H, Davies P. Resveratrol promotes clearance of Alzheimer's disease amyloid-beta peptides. J Biol Chem. 2005 Nov 11;280(45):37377-82.

(58) Martin AR, Villegas I, La CC, de la Lastra CA. Resveratrol, a polyphenol found in grapes, suppresses oxidative damage and stimulates apoptosis during early colonic inflammation in rats. Biochem Pharmacol. 2004 Apr 1;67(7):1399-410.

(59) Martin R. Novel strategy to restore brain cell function. Life Extension. May, 2006:24-31.

(60) Martinez J, Moreno JJ. Effect of resveratrol, a natural polyphenolic compound, on reactive oxygen species and prostaglandin production. Biochem Pharmacol. 2000; 59:865-870.

(61) Mitchell T. Broad-spectrum effects of grape seed extract. Life Extension. July, 2005:32-9.

(62) Mokni M, Limam F, Elkahoui S, Amri M, Aouani E. Strong cardioprotective effect of resveratrol, a red wine polyphenol, on isolated rat

hearts after ischemia/reperfusion injury. Arch Biochem Biophys. 2007 Jan 1;457(1):1-6.

(63) Nielsen M, Ruch RJ, Vang O. Resveratrol reverses tumor-promoter-induced inhibition of gap-junctional intercellular communication. Biochem Biophys Res Commun. 2000; 275:804-809.

(64) Novakovic A, Bukarica LG, Kanjuh V, Heinle H. Potassium channels-mediated vasorelaxation of rat aorta induced by resveratrol. Basic Clin Pharmacol Toxicol. 2006 Nov;99(5):360-4.

(65) Olas B, Wachowicz B. Resveratrol and vitamin C as antioxidants in blood platelets. Thromb Res. 2002 Apr 15;106(2):143-8.

(66) Olas B, Wachowicz B, Saluk-Juszczak J, Zielinski T. Effect of resveratrol, a natural polyphenolic compound, on platelet activation induced by endotoxin or thrombin. Thromb Res. 2002 Aug 15;107(3-4):141-5.

(67) Olas B, Wachowicz B, Majsterek I, et al. Antioxidant properties of trans-3,3',5,5'-tetrahydroxy-4'-methoxystilbene against modification of variety of biomolecules in human blood cells treated with platinum compounds. Nutrition. 2006 Nov;22(11-12):1202-9.

(68) Pace-Asciak CR, Hahn S, Diamandis EP, et al. The red wine phenolics trans-resveratrol and quercetin block human platelet aggregation and eicosanoid synthesis: implications for protection against coronary heart disease. Clin Chim Acta. 1995; 235:207-219.

(69) Paul B, Masih I, Deopujari J, Charpentier C. Occurrence of resveratrol and pterostilbene in age-old darakchasava, an ayurvedic medicine from India. J Ethnopharmacol. 1999; 68:71-76.

(70) Pinto MC, García-Barrado JA, Macías P. Resveratrol is a potent inhibitor of the dioxygenase activity of lipoxygenase. J Agric Food Chem. 1999; 47:4842-4846.

(71) Porcu M, Chiarugi A. The emerging therapeutic potential of sirtuin-interacting drugs: from cell death to lifespan extension. Trends Pharmacol Sci. 2005 Feb;26(2):94-103.

(72) Potter GA, Patterson LH, Wanogho E, Perry PJ, Butler PC, Ijaz T, Ruparelia KC, Lamb JH, Farmer PB, Stanley LA, Burke MD. The cancer preventative agent resveratrol is converted to the anticancer agent piceatannol by the cytochrome P450 enzyme CYP1B1. Br J Cancer. 2002 Mar 4;86(5):774-8.

(73) Prokop J, Abrman P, Seligson AL, Sovak M. Resveratrol and its glycon piceid are stable polyphenols. J Med Food. 2006;9(1):11-4.

(74) Ray PS, Maulik G, Cordis GA, et al. The red wine antioxidant resveratrol protects isolated rat hearts from ischemia reperfusion injury. Free Rad Biol Med. 1999; 27:160-169.

(75) Rezai-Zadeh K, Shytle D, Sun N, et al. Green tea epigallocatechin-3-gallate (EGCG) modulates amyloid precursor protein cleavage and reduces cerebral amyloidosis in Alzheimer transgenic mice. J Neurosci. 2005 Sep 21;25(38):8807-14.

(76) Richard N, Porath D, Radspieler A, Schwager J. Effects of resveratrol, piceatannol, tri-acetoxystilbene, and genistein on the inflammatory response of human peripheral blood leukocytes. Mol Nutr Food Res. 2005 May;49(5):431-42.

(77) Sanders TH, McMichael RW Jr, Hendrix KW. Occurrence of resveratrol in edible peanuts. J Agric Food Chem. 2000; 48:1243-1246.

(78) Savaskan E, Olivieri G, Meier F, et al. Red wine ingredient resveratrol protects from beta-amyloid neurotoxicity. Gerontology. 2003 Nov;49(6):380-3.

(79) Schneider Y, Vincent F, Duranton B, et al. Anti-proliferative effect of resveratrol, a natural component of grapes and wine, on human colonic cancer cells. Cancer Lett. 2000; 158:85-91.

(80) Sharma M, Gupta YK. Chronic treatment with trans resveratrol prevents intracerebroventricular streptozotocin induced cognitive impairment and oxidative stress in rats. Life Sci. 2002 Oct 11;71(21):2489-98.

(81) Sinclair DA. Toward a unified theory of caloric restriction and longevity regulation. Mech Ageing Dev. 2005 Sep;126(9):987-1002.

(82) Soleas GJ, Diamandis EP, Goldberg DM. Resveratrol: A molecule whose time has come? And gone? Clin Biochem. 1997; 30:91-113.

(83) Sovak M. Grape extract, resveratrol, and its analogs: a review. J Med Food. 2001;4(2):93-105.

(84) Stewart JR, Christman KL, O'Brian CA. Effects of resveratrol on the autophosphorylation of phorbol ester-responsive protein kinases. Biochem Pharmacol. 2000; 60:1355-1359.

(85) Subbaramaiah K, Chung WJ, Michaluart P, et al. Resveratrol inhibits cyclooxygenase-2 transcription and activity in phorbol ester-treated human mammary epithelial cells. J Biol Chem. 1998; 273:21875-21882.

(86) Szewczuk and Penning. Mechanism-based inactivation of COX-1 by red wine m-hydroquinones: a structure-activity study. J Nat Prod 67i(11):1777-82 (2004).

(87) Subbaramaiah K, Michaluart P, Chung WJ, et al. Resveratrol inhibits cyclooxygenase-2 transcription in human mammary epithelial cells. Ann NY Acad Sci. 2000; 889:214-223.

(88) Tang W, Eisenbrand G. Chinese Drugs of Plant Origin. Berlin: Springer-Verlag; 1992; 787-791.

(89) Tessitore L, Davit A, Sarotto I, Caderni G. Resveratrol depresses the growth of colorectal aberrant crypt foci by affecting bax and p21CIP expression. Carcinogenesis. 2000; 21:1619-1622.

(90) Tomera JF. Current knowledge of the health benefits and disadvantages of wine consumption. Trends Food Sci Technol. 1999; 10:129-138.

(91) Trincheri NF, Nicotra G, Follo C, Castino R, Isidoro C. Resveratrol induces cell death in colorectal cancer cells by a novel pathway involving lysosomal cathepsin D. Carcinogenesis. 2006 Nov 20.

(92) Tsai SH, Lin-Shiau SY, Lin JK. Suppression of nitric oxide synthase and the down-regulation of the activation of NFkappaB in macrophages by resveratrol. Br J Pharmacol. 1999; 126:673-680.

(93) Valenzano DR, Terzibasi E, Genade T, et al. Resveratrol prolongs lifespan and retards the onset of age-related markers in a short-lived vertebrate. Curr Biol. 2006 Feb 7;16(3):296-300.

(94) Vigna GB, Costantini F, Aldini G, et al. Effect of a standardized grape seed extract on low-density lipoprotein susceptibility to oxidation in heavy smokers. Metabolism. 2003 Oct;52(10):1250-7.

(95) Vinson JA, Proch J, Bose P. MegaNatural((R)) gold grapeseed extract: in vitro antioxidant and in vivo human supplementation studies. J Med Food. 2001;4(1):17-26.

(96) Wagner E. Grape seed extract promotes bone formation. Life Extension. October, 2006:24.

(97) Wang Z, Huang Y, Zou J, et al. Effects of red wine and wine polyphenol resveratrol on platelet aggregation in vivo and in vitro. Int J Mol Med. 2002 Jan;9(1):77-9.

(98) Wang J, Ho L, Zhao Z, et al. Moderate consumption of cabernet sauvignon attenuates abeta neuropathology in a mouse model of Alzheimer's disease. FASEB J. 2006 Nov;20(13):2313-20.

(99) Wood JG, Rogina B, Lavu S, et al. Sirtuin activators mimic caloric restriction and delay ageing in metazoans. Nature. 2004 Aug 5;430(7000):686-9.

(100) Zhang J. Resveratrol inhibits insulin responses in a SirT1-independent pathway. Biochem J. 2006 Aug 1;397(3):519-27.

Chapter 21 - Green Tea References

(1) Song, JM, Lee, KH, Seong, BL, Antiviral effects of catechins in green tea on influenza virus, Antiviral Research, 2005 Nov; 68(2):66-74

(2) Chou CC. Int J Food Microbiol 1999; 48:125-130.
Kansenshogaku Zasshi 1997 Jun; 71(6): 487-94.

Jack F. Bukowski, Harvard Medical School, Science News, August 21, 1999. p. 127.

(3) Alice M. Green tea for remission maintenance in Crohn's disease? Am J Gastroenterol. 1999;94(6):1710.

(4) Blumenthal M, ed. The Complete German Commission E Monographs. Therapeutic Guide to Herbal Medicines. Boston, Mass: Integrative Medicine Communications; 1998:47, 132.

(5) Brinker F. Herb Contraindications and Drug Interactions. 2nd ed. Sandy, OR: Eclectic Medical Publications; 1998:126-129.

(6) Brown MD. Green tea (Camellia sinensis) extract and its possible role in the prevention of cancer. Alt Med Rev. 1999;4(5):360-370.

(7) Bushman JL. Green tea and cancer in humans: a review of the literature. Nutr Cancer. 1998;31(3):151-159.

(8) Craig WJ. Health-promoting properties of common herbs. Am J Clin Nutr. 1999;70(suppl):491S-499S.

(9) Dulloo AG, Duret C, Rohrer D, et al. Efficacy of a green tea extract rich in catechin polyphenols and caffeine in increasing 24-h energy expenditure and fat oxidation in humans. Am J Clin Nutr. 1999;70:1040-1045.

(10) Ernst E, ed. The Desktop Guide to Complementary and Alternative Medicine: An Evidence-Based Approach. Mosby, Edinburgh; 2001:119-121.

(11) Ernst E, Cassileth BR. How useful are unconventional cancer treatments? Eur J Cancer. 1999;35(11):1608-1613.

(12) Fujiki H, Suganuma M, Okabe S, et al. Cancer inhibition by green tea. Mutation Research. 1998;307-310.

(13) Fujiki H, Suganuma M, Okabe S, et al. Mechanistic findings of green tea as cancer preventive for humans. Proc Soc Exp Biol Med. 1999;220(4):225-228.

(14) Gao Yt, McLaughlin JK, Blot WJReduced risk of esophageal cancer associated with green tea consumption. J Natl Cancer Inst. 1994 Jun 1;86(11):855-8.

(15) Geleijnse JM, Launer LJ, Hofman A, Pols HA, Witteman JCM. Tea flavonoids may protect against atherosclerosis: the Rotterdam study. Arch Intern Med. 1999;159:2170-2174.

(16) Gomes A, Vedasiromoni JR, Das M, Sharma RM, Ganguly DK. Anti-hyperglycemic effect of black tea (Camellia sinensis) in rat. J Ethnopharmocolgy. 1995;45:223-226.

(17) Gruenwalkd J, Brendler T, Jaenicke C, scientific eds; Fleming T, chief ed. PDR for Herbal Medicines. 2nd ed. Montvale, NJ:Medical Economics Company; 2000:369-372.

155

(18) Heck AM, DeWitt BA, Lukes AL. Potential interactions between alternative therapies and warfarin. [review]. Am J Health Syst Pharm. 2000 Jul 1;57(13):1221-1227.

(19) Hu J, Nyren O, Wolk A, Bergstrom R, et al. Risk factors for oesophageal cancer in northeast China. Int J Cancer. 1994;57(1):38-46.

(20) Imai K, Suga K, Nagachi K. Cancer-preventive effects of drinking green tea among a Japanese population. Prev Med. 1997;26(6):769-775.

(21) Inoue M, Tajima K, Mizutani M, et al. Regular consumption of green tea and the risk of breast cancer recurrence: follow-up study from the Hospital-based Epidemiologic Research Program at Aichi Cancer Center (HERPACC), Japan. Cancer Lett. 2001;167(2):175-182.

(22) Ji B-T, Chow W-H, Hsing AW, et al. Green tea consumption and the risk of pancreatic and colorectal cancers. Int J Cancer. 1997;70:255-258.

(23) Kaegi E. Unconventional therapies for cancer: 2. Green tea. [Review]. The Task Force on Alternative Therapies of the Canadian Breast Cancer Research Initiative. CMAJ. 1998;158(8):1033-1035.

(24) Katiyar SK, Ahmad N, Mukhtar H. Green tea and skin. Arch Dermatol. 2000;136(8):989-94.

(25) Katiyar SK, Mukhtar H. Tea antioxidants in cancer chemoprevention. [Review]. J Cell Biochem Suppl. 1997;27:59-67.

(26) Kono S, Shinchi K, Ikeda N, Yanai F, Imanishi K. Green tea consumption and serum lipid profiles: a cross-sectional study in northern Kyushu, Japan. Prev Med. 1992 Jul;21(4):526-531.

(27) Kuroda Y, Hara Y. Antimutagenic and anticarcinogenic activity of tea polyphenols. [Review]. Mutat Res. 1999;436(1):69-97.

(28) Low Dog T, Riley D, Carter T. Traditional and alternative therapies for breast cancer. Alt Ther. 2001;7(3):36-47.

(29) Luo M, Kannar K, Wahlqvist ML, O'Brien RC. Inhibition of LDL oxidation by green tea extract. Lancet. 1997 Feb 1;349(9048):360-361.

(30) Luper S. A review of plants used in the treatment of liver disease: part two. Alt Med Rev. 1999;4(3):178-188.

(31) Lyn-Cook BD, Rogers T, Yan Y, Blann EB, Kadlubar FF, Hammons GJ. Chemopreventive effects of tea extracts and various components on human pancreatic and prostate tumor cells in vitro. Nutr Cancer. 1999;35(1):80-86.

(32) McKenna DJ, Hughes K, Jones K. Green tea monograph. Alt Ther. 2000;6(3):61-84.

(33) Miura Y, Chiba T, Tomita I, et al. Tea catechins prevent the development of atherosclerosis in apoprotein E-deficient mice. J Nutr. 2001;131(1):27-32.

(34) Mukhtar H, Ahmad N. Green tea in chemoprevention of cancer. [Review]. Toxicol Sci. 1999;52(2 Suppl):111-117.

(35) Nakachi K, Suemasu K, Suga K, Takeo T, Imai K, Higashi Y. Influence of drinking green tea on breast cancer malignancy among Japanese patients. Jpn J Cancer Res. 1998;89(3):254-261.

(36) Nagata C, Kabuto M, Shimizu H. Association of coffee, green tea, and caffeine intakes with serum concentrations of estradiol and sex hormone-binding globulin in premenopausal Japanese women. Nutr Cancer. 1998;30(1):21-24.

(37) Ohno Y, Aoki K, Obata K, Morrison AS. Case-control study of urinary bladder cancer in metropolitan Nagoya. Natl Cancer Inst Monogr. 1985;69:229-234.

(38) Ohno Y, Wakai K, Genka K, et al. Tea consumption and lung cancer risk: a case-control study in Okinawa, Japan. Jpn J Cancer Res. 1995;86(11):1027-1034.

(39) Pianetti S, Guo S, Kavanagh KT, Sonenshein GE. Green tea polyphenol epigallocatechin-3 gallate inhibits Her-2/neu signaling, proliferation, and transformed phenotype of breast cancer cells. Cancer Res. 2002;62(3):652-655.

(40) Picard D. The biochemistry of green tea polyphenols and their potential application in human skin cancer. Altern Med Rev. 1996;1(1):31-42.

(41) Robbers JE, Tyler VE. Tyler's Herbs of Choice. New York: The Haworth Herbal Press; 1999: 249-250.

(42) Sadzuka Y, Sugiyama T, Hirota. Modulation of cancer chemotherapy by green tea. Clin Cancer Res. 1998;4(1):153-156.

(43) Sano T, Sasako M. Green tea and gastric cancer. N Engl J Med. 2001;344(9):675-676.

(44) Sasazuki S, Kodama H, Yoshimasu K et al. Relation between green tea consumption and the severity of coronary atherosclerosis among Japanese men and women. Ann Epidemiol. 2000;10:401-408.

(45) Setiawan VW, Zhang ZF, Yu GP, et al. Protective effect of green tea on the risks of chronic gastritis and stomach cancer. Int J Cancer. 2001;92(4):600-604.

(46) Shim JH, Kang MG, Kim YH, Roberts C, Lee IP. Chemopreventive effect of green tea (Camellia sinensis) among cigarette smoke. Cancer-Epidemio-Biomarkers-Prev. 1995;Jun; 4(4): 387-91.

157

(47) Shiota S, Shimizu M, Mizushima T, Ito H, et al. Marked reduction in the minimum inhibitory concentration (MIC) of ß-lactams in methicillin-resistant Staphylococcus aureus produced by epicatechin gallate, an ingredient of green tea (Camellia sinensis). Biol. Pharm. Bull. 1999;22(12):1388-1390.

(48) Suganuma M, Okabe S, Kai Y, Sueoka N, et al. Synergistic effects of (-)-epigallocatechin gallate with (-)-epicatechin, sulindac, or tamoxifen on cancer-preventive activity in the human lung cancer cell line PC-9. Cancer Res. 1999;59:44-47.

(49) Suganuma M, Okabe S, Sueoka N, et al. Green tea and cancer chemoprevention. Mutat Res. 1999 Jul 16;428(1-2):339-344.

(50) Sugiyama T, Sadzuka Y. Combination of theanine with doxorubicin inhibits hepatic metastasis of M5076 ovarian sarcoma. Clin Cancer Res. 1999;5:413-416.

(51) Sugiyama T, Sadzuka Y. Enhancing effects of green tea components on the antitumor activity of adriamycin against M5076 ovarian sarcoma. Cancer Lett. 1998;133(1):19-26.

(52) Taylor JR, Wilt VM. Probable antagonism of warfarin by green tea. Ann Pharmacother. 1999;33(4):426-428.
Tewes FJ, Koo LC, Meisgen TJ, Rylander R. Lung cancer risk and mutagenicity of tea. Environ Res. 1990;52(1):23-33.

(53) Thatte U, Bagadey S, Dahanukar S. Modulation of programmed cell death by medicinal plants. [Review]. Cell Mol Biol. 2000;46(1):199-214.

(54) Tsubono Y, Nishino Y, Komatsu S, et al. Green tea and the risk of gastric cancer in Japan. N Engl J Med. 2001;344(9):632-636.

(55) van het Hof KH, de Boer HS, Wiseman SA, Lien N, Westrate JA, Tijburg LB. Consumption of green or black tea does not increase resistance of low-density lipoprotein to oxidation in humans. Am J Clin Nutr. 1997 Nov;66(5):1125-1132.

(56) Wakai K, Ohno Y, Obata K, Aoki K. Prognostic significance of selected lifestyle factors in urinary bladder cancer. Jpn J Cancer Res. 1993 Dec;84(12):1223-1229.

(57) Wang Z, et al. Antimutagenic activity of green tea polyphenols. Mutation Research. 1989;223:273-285.

(58) Wargovich MJ, Woods C, Hollis DM, Zander ME. Herbals, cancer prevention and health. [Review]. J Nutr. 2001;131(11 Suppl):3034S-3036S.

(59) Wei H, Zhang X, Zhao JF, Wang ZY, Bickers D, Lebwohl M. Scavenging of hydrogen peroxide and inhibition of ultraviolet light-induced oxidative DNA damage by aqueous extracts from green and black teas. Free Radic Biol Med. 1999;26(11-12):1427-1435.

(60) Weisburger JH. Tea and health: a historic perspective. Cancer Letters. 1997;114:315-317.

(61) Windridge C. The Fountain of Health. An A-Z of Traditional Chinese Medicine. London, England: Mainstream Publishing; 1994:259.

(62) Yamane T, Nakatani H, Kikuoka N, et al. Inhibitory effects and toxicity of green tea polyphenols for gastrointestinal carcinogenesis. Cancer. 1996;77(8 Suppl):1662-1667.

(63) Yang TT, Koo MW. Hypocholesterolemic effects of Chinese tea. Pharmacol Res. 1997;35(6):505-512.

(64) Yang TTC, Koo MWI. Chinese green tea lowers cholesterol level through an increase in fecal lipid excreiton. Life Sciences. 1999:66:5:411-423.

(65) Yu GP, Hsieh CC, Wang LY, Yu SZ, Li XL, Jin TH. Green-tea consumption and risk of stomach cancer: a population-based case-control study in Shanghai, China. Cancer Causes Control. 1995;6(6):532-538.

(66) Tao P. The inhibitory effects of catechin derivatives on the activities of human immunodeficiency virus reverse transcriptase and DNA polymerases. Chung Kuo 1992; 14:334-38.

(67) Nakane H, Ono K. Differential inhibition of HIV reverse transcriptase and various DNA and RNA polymerases by some catechin derivatives. Nucleic Acids Symp Ser 1989; (21): 115-16.

(68) Hamilton-Miller JM. Antimicrobial properties of tea (Camellia sinensis L.). Antimicro Agents Chemother 1995;39:2375–7.

(69) Chou CC. Int J Food Microbiol 1999; 48:125-130.
Interview with Milton Schiffenbauer of Pace University.
Kansenshogaku Zasshi 1997 Jun; 71(6): 487-94.

(70) Jack F. Bukowski, Harvard Medical School, Science News, August 21, 1999. p. 127.

(71) United States Patent 7175987, Compositions and methods for treatment of herpes, US Patent Issued on Feb. 13, 2007

(72) HTLV-1 provirus load in peripheral blood lymphocytes of HTLV-1 carriers is diminished by green tea drinking. Cancer Sci. 2004 Jul;95(7):596-601

(73) Inhibition of adenovirus infection and adenain by green tea catechins. Antiviral Res. 2003 Apr;58(2):167-73

(74) Inhibition of Epstein-Barr virus lytic cycle by (-)-epigallocatechin gallate. Biochem Biophys Res Commun. 2003 Feb 21;301(4):1062-8

(75) Antiviral properties of prodelphinidin B-2 3'-O-gallate from green tea leaf. Antivir Chem Chemother. 2002 Jul;13(4):223-9

(76) Additional inhibitory effect of tea extract on the growth of influenza A and B viruses in MDCK cells. Microbiol Immunol. 2002;46(7):491-4

(77) Protective effects of green tea extracts (polyphenon E and EGCG) on human cervical lesions. Eur J Cancer Prev 2003 Oct;12(5):383-90

(78) Polyphenolic antioxidant (-)-epigallocatechin-3-gallate from green tea as a candidate anti-HIV agent. AIDS. 2002 Apr 12;16(6):939-41

(79) Inhibitory Effects of Polyphenolic Catechins from Chinese Green Tea on HIV Reverse Transcriptase Activity. J Biomed Sci. 1994 Jun;1(3):163-166

(80) Inhibition of rotavirus and enterovirus infections by tea extracts. Jpn J Med Sci Biol. 1991 Aug;44(4):181-6

(81) Epigallocatechin gallate, the main polyphenol in green tea, binds to the T-cell receptor, CD4: Potential for HIV-1 therapy. J Allergy Clin Immunol. 2006 Dec;118(6):1369-74. Epub 2006 Oct 13

(82) EGCG mitigates neurotoxicity mediated by HIV-1 proteins gp120 and Tat in the presence of IFN-gamma: role of JAK/STAT1 signaling and implications for HIV-associated dementia. Brain Res. 2006 Dec 6;1123(1):216-25. Epub 2006 Oct 31

(83) How can (-)-epigallocatechin gallate from green tea prevent HIV-1 infection? Mechanistic insights from computational modeling and the implication for rational design of anti-HIV-1 entry inhibitors. J Phys Chem B. 2006 Feb 16;110(6):2910-7

(84) Inhibitory effects of (-)-epigallocatechin gallate on the life cycle of human immunodeficiency virus type 1 (HIV-1). Antiviral Res. 2002 Jan;53(1):19-34

(85) http://www.greenteahaus.com

(86) Cao J, Bai X, Zhao Y, Liu J, Zhou D, Fang S, Jia M, Wu J - "The relationship of fluorosis and brick tea drinking in Chinese Tibetans" Environ Health Perspect 104(12):1340-3 (1996)

(87) Cao J, Zhao Y, Liu J - "Brick tea consumption as the cause of dental fluorosis among children from Mongol, Kazak and Yugu populations in China" Food Chem Toxicol 35(8):827-33 (1997)

(88) Cao J, Zhao Y, Liu JW - "Safety evaluation and fluorine concentration of Pu'er brick tea and Bianxiao brick tea" Food Chem Toxicol 36(12):1061-3 (1998)

(89) Sergio Gomez S, Weber A, Torres C - "Fluoride content of tea and amount ingested by children" Odontol Chil 37(2):251-5 (1989)

(90) Gulati P, Singh V, Gupta MK, Vaidya V, Dass S, Prakash S - "Studies on the leaching of fluoride in tea infusions" Sci Total Environ.138(1-3):213-21 (1993)

(91) Chan J.T.; Koh, S.H. -"Fluoride content in caffeinated, decaffeinated and herbal teas" Caries Res 30(1):88-92 (1996)

(92) Chan J.T.; Yip, T.T.; Jeske, A.H. - "The role of caffeinated beverages in dental fluorosis" Med Hypotheses 33(1):21-2 (1990)

(93) Schmidt, C.W.; Leuschke, W. - "Fluoride content of deciduous teeth after regular intake of black tea" Dtsch Stomatol 40(10):441 (1990)

(94) Wei, S.H.; Hattab, F.N., Mellberg, J.R. - "Concentration of fluoride and selected other elements in teas" Nutrition 5(4):237-40 (1989)
(95) Nabrzyski M, Gajewska R - "Aluminium and fluoride in hospital daily diets and in teas" Z Lebensm Unters Forsch 201(4):307-10 (1995)

(96) Koch K. R., Pougnet B., De Villiers S.: "Increased urinary excretion of Al after drinking tea" Nature 333 (May 12, 1988)

(97) Zeyuan D, Bingying T, Xiaolin L, Jinming H, Yifeng C- "Effect of green tea and black tea on the metabolisms of mineral elements in old rats." Biol Trace Elem Res 65(1):75-86 (1998)

(98) Frech, F.- "Alzheimer's Disease:Solving The Mystery". In a speech before a health care workers conference at Shawnee-Mission, Kansas, Medical Centre, September 14, 1993. (Population Renewal Office, 36 West 59th Street, Kansas City, MO 64113-1246)

(99) Isaacson, R - "Rat studies link brain cell damage with aluminum and fluoride in water" State Univ. of New York, Binghampton, NY 1-607-777-2000 (Wall Street Journal article by Marilyn Chase; Oct.28, 1992, p.B-6)

(100) Strunecká A, Patocka J - "Aluminum and fluoride: a new, deadly duo in Alzheimer's Disease" Cesk Fysiol 48(1):9-15 (1999)

(101) http://www.bruha.com/pfpc/html/green_tea___.html

(102) http://www.umm.edu/altmed/articles/green-tea-000255.htm

Chapter 22 - Olive Leaf Extract References

(1) Fehri B, Aiache JM, Memmi A, Korbi S, Yacoubi MT, Mrad S, Lamaison JL. Hypotension, hypoglycemia and hypouricemia recorded after repeated administration of aqueous leaf extract of Olea europaea L. J Pharm Belg . 1994;49:101-8.

(2) Khayyal MT, el-Ghazaly MA, Abdallah DM, Nassar NN, Okpanyi SN, Kreuter MH. Blood pressure lowering effect of an olive leaf extract (Olea europaea) in L-NAME induced hypertension in rats. Arzneimittelforschung . 2002;52:797-802.

(3) Ribeiro Rde A, Fiuza de Melo MM, De Barros F, Gomes C, Trolin G. Acute antihypertensive effect in conscious rats produced by some medicinal plants used in the state of Sao Paulo. J Ethnopharmacol . 1986;15:261-9.

161

(4) Zarzuelo A, Duarte J, Jimenez J, Gonzalez M, Utrilla MP. Vasodilator effect of olive leaf. Planta Med . 1991;57:417-9.

(5) Katsiki M, Chondrogianni N, Chinou I, Rivett AJ, Gonos ES. The olive constituent oleuropein exhibits proteasome stimulatory properties in vitro and confers life span extension of human embryonic fibroblasts. Rejuvenation Research. 2007;10(2):157-172.

(6) Puel C, Mathey J, Agalias A, Kati-Coulibaly S, Mardon J, Obled C, Davicco MJ, Lebecque P, Horcajada MN, Skaltsounis AL, Coxam V. Dose-response study of effect of oleuropein, an olive oil polyphenol, in an ovariectomy/inflammation experimental model of bone loss in the rat. Clin Nutr. 2006 May 30

(7) De Laurentis N, et al. Flavonoids from leaves of Olea europaea L. cultivars. Ann Pharm Fr. 1998;56(6):268-73.
Ficarra P, et al. HPLC analysis of oleuropein and some flavonoids in leaf and bud of Olea europaea L. Farmaco. Jun1991;46(6):803-15.

(8) PDR for Herbal Medicines, 2nd edition. Montvale, NJ: Medical Economics Company; 2000:557.

(9) American Herbal Products Association. Use of Marker Compounds in Manufacturing and Labeling Botanically Derived Dietary Supplements. Silver Spring, MD: American Herbal Products Association; 2001.

(10) Ferro-Luzzi A, et al. Changing the Mediterranean diet: effects on blood lipids. Am J Clin Nutr. Nov1984;40(5):1027-37.

(11) Kushi LH, et al. Health implications of Mediterranean diets in light of contemporary knowledge. 2. Meat, wine, fats, and oils. Am J Clin Nutr. Jun1995;61(6 Suppl):1416S-1427S.

(12) Visoli F, et al. Oleuropein protects low density lipoprotein from oxidation. Life Sciences. 1994;55:1965-71.

(13) Soret MG. Antiviral activity of calcium elenolate on parainfluenza infection of hamsters. Antimicrobial Agents and Chemotherapy. 1969;9:160-66.

(14) Bisignano G, et al. On the in-vitro antimicrobial activity of oleuropein and hydroxytyrosol. J Pharm Pharmacol. Aug1999;51(8):971-4.

(15) Petkov V, Manolov P. Pharmacological analysis of the iridoid oleuropein. Drug Res. 1972;22(9):1476-86.
Juven B, et al. Studies on the mechanism of the antimicrobial action of oleuropein. J Appl Bact. 1972;35:559.

(16) Visioli F, et al. Oleuropein, the bitter principle of olives, enhances nitric oxide production by mouse macrophages. Life Sci. 1998;62(6):541-6.

(17) Renis HE. In vitro antiviral activity of calcium elenolate. Antimicrob. Agents Chemother. 1970;167-72.

162

(18) Heinze JE, et al. Specificity of the antiviral agent calcium elenolate. Antimicrob Agents Chemother. Oct1975;8(4):421-5.

(19) Renis HE. Inactivation of myxoviruses by calcium elenolate. Antimicrob Agents Chemother. Aug1975;8(2):194-9.

(20) Hirschman SZ. Inactivation of DNA polymerases of murine leukaemia viruses by calcium elenolate. Nat New Biol. Aug1972;238(87):277-9.

(21) Soret MG. Antiviral activity of calcium elenolate on parainfluenza infection of hamsters. Antimicrob Agents Chemother. 1969;9:160-6.

(22) Renis HE. In vitro antiviral activity of calcium elenolate. Antimicrob Agents Chemother. 1970;167-72.
Zarzuelo A, et al. Vasodilator effect of olive leaf. Planta Med. Oct1991;57(5):417-9.

(23) Visioli F, et al. The effect of minor constituents of olive oil on cardiovascular disease: new findings. Nutr Rev. May1998;56(5 Pt 1):142-7.

(24) Giugliano D. Dietary antioxidants for cardiovascular prevention. Nutr Metab Cardiovasc Dis. Feb2000;10(1):38-44.

(25) Visioli F, et al. Oleuropein protects low density lipoprotein from oxidation. Life Sci. 1994;55(24):1965-71.

(26) Petroni A, et al. Inhibition of platelet aggregatiion and eicosanoid production by phenolic components of olive oil. Thromb Res. Apr1995;78(2)151-60.

(27) Hansen K, et al. Isolation of an angiotensin converting enzyme (ACE) inhibitor from olea europaea and olea lacea. Phytomedicine. 1996;2:319-325.

(28) Bennani-Kabchi N, et al. Effects of Olea europea var. oleaster leaves in hypercholesterolemic insulin-resistant sand rats. Therapie. Nov1999;54(6):717-23.

(29) Gonzalez M, et al. Hypoglycemic activity of olive leaf. Planta Medica. 1992;58:513-515.

(30) Chimi H, et al. Inhibition of iron toxicity in rat hepatocyte culture by natural phenolic compounds. Tox In Vitro. 1995;9:695-702.

(31) Pieroni A, et al. In vitro anti-complementary activity of flavonoids from olive (Olea europaea L.) leaves. Pharmazie. Oct1996;51(10):765-8.

(32) PDR for Herbal Medicines, 2nd ed. Montvale, NJ: Medical Economics Company; 2000:557.

(33) Martinez A, et al. Identification of a 36-kDa olive-pollen allergen by in vitro and in vivo studies. Allergy. Jun1999;54(6):584-92.

(34) Cherif S, Rahal N, Haouala M, et al. A clinical trial of a titrated Olea extract in the treatment of essential arterial hypertension. J Pharm Belg . 1996;51:69-71.

(35) Walker, Morton MD. Natures Antibiotic: Olive Leaf Extract, Kensington Books, New York, 1997. pps. 65-68, 39, 149.

(36) Rodriguez MM, Perez J, Ramos-Cormenzana A, Martinez J. Effect of extracts obtained from olive oil mill waste waters on Bacillus megaterium ATCC 33085. Journal of Applied Bacteriology. 1988; 64:219-26.

(37) Tassou CC, Nychas GJE, Board RG. Effect of Phenolic Compounds and Oleuropein on the Germination of Bacillus cereus T Spores. Biotechnology and Applied Biochemistry. 1991; 13:231-37.

(38) Bisignano G, Tomaino A, Lo Cascio R, Crisafi G, Uccella N, Saija A. On the In-Vitro Antimicrobial Activity of Oleuropein and Hydroxytyrosol. J. Pharm. Pharmacol. 1999; 51: 971-74.

(39) Nychas GJE, Tassou SC, Board RG. Phenolic extract from olives: inhibition of Staphylococcus aureus. Letters in Applied Microbiology. 1990; 10: 217-220.

(40) Heinze JE, Hale AH, Carl PL. Specificity of the Antiviral Agent Calcium Elenolate. Antimicrobial Agents and Chemotherapy. 1975; 8(4):421-25.

(41) Hanbury D. On the febrifuge properties of the olive (Olea europea, L.), Pharmaceutical Journal of Provincial Transactions, pp. 353-354, 1854.

(42) Cruess WV, and Alsberg CL, The bitter glucoside of the olive. J Amer. Chem. Soc. 1934; 56:2115-7.

(43) Veer WLC et al. A Compound isolated from Europea. Recueil,1957; 76:839-40.

Chapter 23 - Omega-3 Fatty Acids References

(1) Vegetarian Society, Information Sheet on Omega 3 fats http://www.vegsoc.org/info/omega3.html

(2) Bang HO, Dyerberg J, Horne N. The composition of food consumed by Greenland Eskimos. Acta Med Scand 1976;200:69-73

(3) Owen PA. Coronary thrombosis. Its mechanism and possible prevention by linolenic acid. Ann Intern Med 1965;62:167-84

(4) Billman GE, Hallaq H, Leaf A. Prevention of ischemic-induced ventricular fibrillation by n-3 fatty acids. Proc Natl Acad Sci USA 1994;91:4427-30

(5) Kleiger RE, Miller JP, Bigger JT, Moss AJ, et al. Decreased heart rate variability and its association with increased mortality after acute acute myocardial infarction. Am J Cardiol 1987;59:256-62

(6) Christensen JH, Christensen MS, Dyerberg J, Schmidt EB. Heart rate variability and fatty acid content of blood cell membranes: a dose-response study with n-3 fatty acids. Am J Clin Nutr 1999;70:331-7

(7) Hu FB, Stampfer MJ, Manson JE, et al. Dietary intake of linolenic acid and risk of fatal IHD among women. Am J Clin Nutr 1999;69:890-7

(8) Burr ML, Fehily AM, Gilbert JF, et al. Effects of changes in fat, fish, and fibre intakes on death and myocardial infarction: diet and reinfarction trial (DART). Lancet 1989;2:757-61

(9) Nair SSD, Leitch JW, Falconer J, Garg ML. Prevention of cardiac arrhythmia by dietary (n-3) polyunsaturated fatty acid and their mechanism of action. J Nutr 1997;127:383-93

(10) de Lorgeril M, Renaud S, Mamelle N, et al. Mediterranean alpha-linolenic acid-rich diet in secondary prevention of coronary artery heart disease. Lancet 1994;343:1454-9

(11) Woodman RJ, Mori TA, Burke V, Puddey IB, Watts GF, Beilin LJ. Effects of purified eicosapentaenoic and docosahexaenoic acids on glycemic control, blood pressure, and serum lipids in type 2 diabetic patients with treated hypertension. Am J Clin Nutr 2002;76:1007-15.

(12) Howe PR. Dietary fats and hypertension. Focus on fish oil. Ann N Y Acad Sci 1997;827:339-52.

(13) Morris MC, Sacks F, Rosner B. Does fish oil lower blood pressure? A meta-analysis of controlled trials. Circulation 1993;88:523-33.

(14) Appel LJ, Miller ER 3d, Seidler AJ, Whelton PK. Does supplementation of diet with 'fish oil' reduce blood pressure? A meta-analysis of controlled clinical trials. Arch Intern Med 1993;153:1429-38.

(15) Kremer JM, Lawrence DA, Jubiz W, DiGiacomo R, Rynes R, Bartholomew LE, et al. Dietary fish oil and olive oil supplementation in patients with rheumatoid arthritis. Clinical and immunologic effects. Arthritis Rheum 1990;33:810-20.

(16) Cleland LG, French JK, Betts WH, Murphy GA, Elliott MJ. Clinical and biochemical effects of dietary fish oil supplements in rheumatoid arthritis. J Rheumatol 1988;15:1471-5.

(17) Volker D, Fitzgerald P, Major G, Garg M. Efficacy of fish oil concentrate in the treatment of rheumatoid arthritis. J Rheumatol 2000;27:2343-6.

(18) Lau CS, Morley KD, Belch JJ. Effects of fish oil supplementation on non-steroidal anti-inflammatory drug requirement in patients with mild rheumatoid arthritis-a double-blind placebo controlled study. Br J Rheumatol 1993;32:982-9.

(19) James MJ, Cleland LG. Dietary n-3 fatty acids and therapy for rheumatoid arthritis. Semin Arthritis Rheum 1997;27:85-97.

(20) Green, V.A., K.A. Pituch, J. Itchon, A. Choi, M. O'Reilly, J. Sigafoos, "Internet survey of treatments used by parents of children with autism," Res Dev Disabil, 2006, 27(1):70-84.

(21) Young, G., and J. Conquer. 2005. "Omega-3 fatty acids and neuropsychiatric disorders." Reprod.Nutr.Dev 45(1):1-28.

(22) Genuis, S.J.a.G.K.S. 2006. "Time for an oil check: the role of essential omega-3 fatty acids in maternal and pediatric health." Journal of Perinatology 26:359-365.

(23) Richardson, A.J. 2006. "Omega-3 fatty acids in ADHD and related neurodevelopmental disorders." Int.Rev.Psychiatry 18(2):155-172.

(24) Richardson, A.J., and M.A. Ross. 2000. "Fatty acid metabolism in neurodevelopmental disorder: a new perspective on associations between attention-deficit/hyperactivity disorder, dyslexia, dyspraxia and the autistic spectrum." Prostaglandins Leukot.Essent.Fatty Acids 63(1-2):1-9.

(25) Bell, J.G., et al. 2004. "Essential fatty acids and phospholipase A2 in autistic spectrum disorders." Prostaglandins Leukot.Essent.Fatty Acids 71(4):201-204.

(26) Johnson, S.M., and E. Hollander. 2003. "Evidence that eicosapentaenoic acid is effective in treating autism." J Clin Psychiatry 64(7):848-849.

(27) Simopoulos AP, Cleland LG (eds): "omega-6/omega-3 Essential Fatty Acid Ratio: The Scientific Evidence." *World Rev Nutr Diet*. Basel, Karger, 2003, Vol 92.

(28) Okuyama H. High n-6 to n-3 ratio of dietary fatty acids rather than serum cholesterol as a major risk factor for coronary heart disease. *Eur J Lipid Sci Technol*. 2001; 103:418-22.

(29) Simopoulos AP, Leaf A, Salem Jr N. Statement on the essentiality of and recommended dietary intakes for omega-6 and omega-3 fatty acids. Prostaglandins, Leukotrienes and Essential Fatty Acids 2000;63:119-121.

(30) Erasmus, Udo, Fats and Oils. 1986. Alive books, Vancouver, ISBN 0-920470-16-5 p. 263 (round-number ratio within ranges given.)

(31) Essential Fats in Food Oils, NIH page - http://efaeducation.nih.gov/sig/esstable.html

(32) W.E.M. Lands (1992). Biochemistry and physiology of n-3 fatty acids. *FASEB J* 6: 2530-2536

(33) Kohn A, Gitelman J, Inbar M. Unsaturated free fatty acids inactivate animal enveloped viruses. Arch Virol. 1980;66(4):301-7.

(34) Bang, HO, Dyerberg, J, and Hjorne N. Acta Med Scand, 200: 69-73, 1976.

(35) Carroll KK. Lipids, 1992.

166

(36) Reddy BS. Lipids, 1992.

(37) Rose, DP and Connolly, JM. Lipids, 1992.

(38) Roebuck, BD. Lipids, 1992.

(39) Booyens, J. IRCS Medical Science, 14: 396, 1986.

(40) Shao, Y, Pardini, L and Pardini, RS. Lipids, 1995.

(41) Aronson WJ, Glaspy JA, Reddy ST, Reese D, Heber D, Bagga D. Modulation of omega-3/omega-6 polyunsaturated ratios with dietary fish oils in men with prostate cancer. Urology. 2001;58(2):283-288.

(42) Danao-Camara TC, Shintani TT. The dietary treatment of inflammatory arthritis: case reports and review of the literature. Hawaii Med J. 1999;58(5):126-13

(43) de Deckere EAM. Possible beneficial effect of fish and fish n-3 polyunsaturated fatty acids in breast and colorectal cancer. Eur J Cancer Prev. 1999;8:213-221.

(44) Griffini P, Fehres O, Klieverik L, et al. Dietary omega-3 polyunsaturated fatty acids promote colon carcinoma metastasis in rat liver. Can Res. 1998;58(15):3312-3319.

(45) Terry P, Lichtenstein P, Feychting M, Ahlbom A, Wolk A. Fatty fish consumption and risk of prostate cancer. *Lancet*. 2001;357(9270):1764-1766.

(46) Tsai W-S, Nagawa H, Kaizaki S, Tsuruo T, Muto T. Inhibitory effects of n-3 polyunsaturated fatty acids on sigmoid colon cancer transformants. *J Gastroenterol*. 1998;33:206-212.

(47) http://www.fda.gov/fdac/features/2003/503_fats.html

(48) H Thormar, C E Isaacs, H R Brown, M R Barshatzky and T Pessolano, Inactivation of enveloped viruses and killing of cells by fatty acids and monoglycerides, Antimicrob Agents Chemother. 1987 January; 31(1): 27-31

(49) United States Patent 4,841,023 Horowitz June 20, 1989

Where to Order this Book

(1) You can order online from Amazon.com at:

http://www.amazon.com

Search for this book by title or by the ISBN number:

ISBN-13: 978-1-884979-05-7
ISBN-10: 1-884979-05-x

(2) For wholesale or bookstore orders, go to Ingram Book Group

http://www.ingrampublisherservices.com/retailer/default.asp

One Ingram Blvd.
P.O. Box 3006
LaVergne, TN 37086-1986

(866) 400-5351

Retailer@ingrampublisherservices.com

_____

For all other inquiries, contact the publisher by logging onto the website and using the contact form.

Published by: Clear Springs Press, LLC
             Yelm, WA   U.S.A.
http://www.clspress.com/contact.html